Diagnosis and Treatment in Rheumatology

Authored by

Małgorzata Wisłowska

Rheumatology and Internal Diseases Department CSK MSWiA, Wołowska st, Poland

Diagnosis and Treatment in Rheumatology

Author: Małgorzata Wisłowska

ISBN (Online): 978-1-68108-655-2

ISBN (Print): 978-1-68108-656-9

© 2018, Bentham eBooks imprint.

Published by Bentham Science Publishers – Sharjah, UAE. All Rights Reserved.

General:

1. Any dispute or claim arising out of or in connection with this License Agreement or the Work (including non-contractual disputes or claims) will be governed by and construed in accordance with the laws of the U.A.E. as applied in the Emirate of Dubai. Each party agrees that the courts of the Emirate of Dubai shall have exclusive jurisdiction to settle any dispute or claim arising out of or in connection with this License Agreement or the Work (including non-contractual disputes or claims).

2. Your rights under this License Agreement will automatically terminate without notice and without the need for a court order if at any point you breach any terms of this License Agreement. In no event will any delay or failure by Bentham Science Publishers in enforcing your compliance with this License Agreement constitute a waiver of any of its rights.

3. You acknowledge that you have read this License Agreement, and agree to be bound by its terms and conditions. To the extent that any other terms and conditions presented on any website of Bentham Science Publishers conflict with, or are inconsistent with, the terms and conditions set out in this License Agreement, you acknowledge that the terms and conditions set out in this License Agreement shall prevail.

Bentham Science Publishers Ltd.
Executive Suite Y - 2
PO Box 7917, Saif Zone
Sharjah, U.A.E.
Email: subscriptions@benthamscience.org

**BENTHAM
SCIENCE**

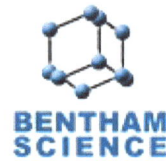

CONTENTS

FOREWORD

This book has been written to summarize all key rheumatic diseases into one clear and concise reference text, which includes current treatment and statistics in the field of rheumatology.

This book presents all up to date information that is easily accessible by medical professionals and students.

Emphasis has been placed on precise and early diagnosis of diseases, as well as reports and findings covering current treatments used, as well as alternative therapies which are being investigated.

Each chapter has a clear heading and follows a logical pattern of disease definition, clinical features, epidemiology, pathology, diagnosis and treatment, making it ideal to find information quickly and effectively.

Students may find this book helpful, as the information is presented in facts, short texts and tables, so that the main features of each diseases are highlighted.

This textbook is factual and an easy read, making it ideal in understanding the field of rheumatology, which was after all, the main aim in composing this book.

Prof. Ireneusz Kotela PhD. MD.
Head of Othopedics and Traumatology Department CSK MSWiA
Warsaw
Poland

PREFACE

Rheumatology in the 21st century uses current cellular, biochemical and immunologic techniques to explain the etiology of rheumatic diseases. While it is unlikely that molecular biology will differentiate rheumatic diseases into subsets based on their etiology, the genome revolution does provide us with new diagnostic tools, which are already beginning to have an impact.

In the past 20 years there have been substantial advances in the field of rheumatology in the management of rheumatoid arthritis (RA), spondyloarthritis (SpA), psoriatic arthritis (PsA), systemic lupus erythematosus (SLE) and vasculitis. Following the introduction of the treatment recommendations for RA in 2016 by the European League Against Rheumatism (EULAR), and the introduction of biological agents and targeted synthetic agents in the management of RA, there is a need to consider the selection of the most appropriate therapy for an individual patient and to review how and when to switch treatments in those patients who do not show an optimal response.

CONSENT FOR PUBLICATION

Not applicable.

CONFLICT OF INTEREST

The author declares no conflict of interest, financial or otherwise.

ACKNOWLEDGEMENT

Declare none.

Prof. Małgorzata Wisłowska PhD. MD.
Head of Rheumatology and Internal Diseases Department CSK MSWiA
Warsaw
Poland

Introduction

Currently, in the field of rheumatology, cellular, biochemical and immunologic techniques are used to explain the etiology of rheumatic diseases. With the use of genomic revolution techniques, we are provided with new diagnostic tools which are expanding and changing the field of rheumatology.

Substancial advances have been made in the management of RA, SpA, PsA, SLE and vasculitis. The big progress in therapy of these diseases is a therapy called "biologic". In RA include tumor necrosis factor (TNF) blockers, monoclonal antibody that inhibits IL-6 receptor signalling, ritiximab (an anti-CD20 chimeric monoclonal antibody that induces B cell and plasmablast depletion), abatacept (an inhibitor of costimulatory signals during antigen presentation). The targeted synthetic agents are the inhibitors of the Janus kinase, the signal transducer and activator of transduction (JAK-STAT) pathway. This pathway is the signaling target of a multitude of cytokines, including INFγ, IL-2, IL-4, IL-6, IL-7, IL-10, IL-12 and IL-15, all of which have biologically significant roles in rheumatoid synovial inflammation.

We are now able to consider the most appropriate therapy for individual patients and to review treatments, potentially switching and adjusting it in patients who do not show optimal responses.

In PsA besides TNFα inhibitors, new options for treatment are inhibitor IL-17 (ixekizumab or sekukinumab), ustekinumab – a fully human IgG 1 k monoclonal antibody that binds to the common p40 subunit shared by interleukins 12 and 23, and apremilast – a phosphodiesterase inhibitor.

Belimumab, a fully human monoclonal antibody that inhibits B-lymphocyte stimulator BLYSS, was approved for the treatment of lupus. There are also a number of other novel therapies in development. The clinical data for these agents and their impact on the management of lupus is an important topic.

Rituximab has been found to be an alternative to cyclophosphomide (CYC) in the treatment of vasculitis for remission induction in newly diagnosed patients with severe ANCA-associated vasculitis. Rituximab in combination with glucocorticoids is used for the treatment of granulomatosis with polyangiitis (GPA) and microscopic polyangiitis (MPA), two forms of ANCA-associated vasculitis. Tocilizumab is a good option to treatment patients with Takayashu arteritis and giant cell arteritis.

Proteomics and genomics offer new opportunities to identify biomarkers that provide surrogates of disease activity and response to therapy. MicroRNAs are small, imperfectly paired, double-stranded RNAs expressed in all cells regulating the expression of hundreds of genes by inhibiting the translation and promoting the degradation of messenger RNAs. MicroRNAs act as master regulators of how a cell responds to changes in its environment, including growth factors and environmental stressors.

The majority of rheumatic diseases have a complex etiology where multiple genetic and environmental effects interact to cause disease. Many rheumatic conditions are associated with human leukocyte antigen (HLA) class II or class I locus alleles, suggesting an immune-mediated component to these diseases.

The pathogenesis of rheumatic diseases involves inflammatory and immune-mediated processes mediated by multiple cell types, like T and B lymphocytes, monocytes/macrophages, neutrophils, and mast cells. Surface receptors on these cells bind to soluble factors, antigens, or other cellular components, that cause these cells to become activated. After activation these cells produce a myriad of soluble factors to recruit and activate additional immune and inflammatory cells. Within of cells after engagement of a cell surface receptor, triggers a cascade of intracellular biochemical events, that couple the receptor signals from the cell surface to the nucleus for modulation of gene transcription *via* a process called signal transduction. Receptor-mediated signal transduction is a basic cellular process essential for communicating events at the cell surface.

The immune system must function to achieve an equilibrium that will favor host defense against foreign pathogens, while protecting host tissues from collateral damage. The immune system is divided into the older immune system (the innate immune system) and the more sophisticated system (the adaptive immune system). Pro-inflammatory (*i.e.* IL-1, IL-6, TNFα, IL-17) and anti-inflammatory (*i.e.* IL-10, TGFβ) cytokines (small proteins released from cells) and chemokines (chemotactic cytokines) provide molecular signals for communication between cells, and play significant roles in sustaining and regulating inflammatory reactions.

Innate immunity detects and responds to a variety of microorganism-derived molecular components, which are not expressed in the host. The innate immune cells are polymorphonuclear leucocytes, monocyte/macrophages, dendritic cells, mast cells and natural killer (NK) cells. Receptor systems for microbial recognition are functionally categorized into three classes according to function: signaling, internalizing and soluble receptors. Signaling receptors such as Toll-like receptors trigger signaling pathways for activating immune response genes. Internalizing receptors integrate micro-organisms and degrade or process them for presentation to T cells. Soluble receptors opsonize micro-organisms and make them components for internalization. This system is activated when it is recognized by receptor's molecular patterns, that are expressed by bacteria as lipopolysaccharides (LPS) or double-stranded RNA, which are only present in bacteria and retroviruses. The activation of innate immune cells occurs mainly through recognition of microbial products called PAMPs (pathogen-associated molecular patterns), by receptors called PRRs (pattern recognition receptors), of which the best known family is called the TLRs (toll-like receptors). PAMPS induce cellular activation, production of acute inflammatory mediators (enzymes, prostaglandins, nitric oxide, free radicals) and up-regulate molecules on the surface of antigen-presenting cells that activate the adaptive immune system. The innate immune system is a simple and immediate response, which can eliminate external attackers rapidly by phagocytosis of the "attackers".

The adaptive immune system consists of T and B cells. They produce a large array of T cell receptors and immunoglobulins using somatic gene recombination. When first encountered the adaptive immune response is slow in responding to an invader, because the T and B cells first need to become activated in draining lymph nodes. The cells can recognize pathogens in a very specific manner, and have immunological memory. The adaptive immune cells (lymphocytes) require training that occurs in the central lymphoid organs (thymus and bone marrow), followed by activation in the peripheral lymphoid organs (spleen, bone marrow, mucous membranes). Maturation of T cells (in the thymus) and B cells (in the bone marrow) is a fundamental step designed to select "good" lymphocytes that are highly efficient in destroying pathogens, but incapable of reacting against self-tissue/host proteins. Therefore, these lymphocytes must be tolerant; otherwise, an autoimmune disease will occur. The major antigen presenting cell for T cells are the dendritic cell and macrophages, and integrate the innate and adaptive immune systems. After an exposure to bacteria or a virus, dendritic cells undergo a process of maturation to become cells capable of activating lymphocytes. This requires the phagocytosis of the foreign pathogen and sensing of microbe associated molecules PAMPs, by specific receptors PRRs. After arrival in the lymphoid organ, the dendritic cell or T cells activate by presenting microbial antigen in the context of human leucocyte antigen (HLA) in conjunction with a second signal, a co-stimulation provided through CD80/CD86-CD28 interaction, where CD80/86 are expressed by the dendritic cells and CD28 by the T cell.

An important part of the adaptive immune system fighting and invading pathogens is mediated by antibodies (humoral immunity). The production of antibodies (glycoproteins), that can bind and neutralize pathogens, and their toxic products in the extracellular spaces of the body, is one of the most important functions of B cells. Antibodies bind to the molecules of pathogens, that induce an immune reaction and are able to activate other molecules of the immune system (such as the complement system) in order to eradicate the pathogen. Antibodies are able to bind antigen in order to neutralize or opsonize antigens for lysis by complement. Antibodies can exert several different effector functions: neutralization of viruses or toxic products from pathogens, complement-mediated lysis of microorganisms, opsonization of microorganisms for phagocytosis, and antibody-dependent cellular cytotoxicity (ADCC). Recognition of antibody-antigen complexes is dependent by the Fc-receptors. B cells often need help from CD4+ T helper (Th) cells for optimal memory. The cells come in different subsets (Th1, Th2, Th17 and Treg cells) that are generated from naïve precursor T cells. Th1 cells function to activate macrophages in ways that enhance microbial killing.Th1 cells are characterized by the profile of cytokines they produce INFγ. Th2 cells have evolved to participate in responses against parasitic infestation, and secrete cytokines such as IL-4, IL-5 and IL-10. IL-4 preferentially induces the synthesis of IgG4 and IgE. Th2 cells play key roles in atopic and allergic disease. Th17 cells participate in host defense against fungal infections, such as Candida. Th17 contribute to organ specific autoimmunity, including inflammatory arthritis and demyelinating disease. T specific populations of CD4+ T-cells (Tregs or CD4+CD25+) exert regulatory function. This population is necessary to maintain homeostasis of the immune system by preventing the activation of self-reactive lymphoid populations.

An immune deficiency may promote the emergence of serious infection or neoplastic disease. A "badly adapted" immune reaction may trigger allergic, inflammatory and autoimmune disease.

INFLAMMATION

The cardinal signs of inflammation are pain (*dolor*), redness (*rubor*), swelling (*tumor*) and loss of function (*function laesa*). Enlarged capillaries that result from vasodilatation cause redness (*erythema*), and an increase in tissue temperature. Increased capillary permeability allows for an influx of fluid and cells, contributing to swelling (*edema*). Phagocytic cells attracted to the site release lytic enzymes, damaging healthy cells. An accumulation of dead cells and fluid forms pus, while mediators released by phagocytic cells stimulate nerves and cause pain.

Inflammation is the primary process by which the body attacks and destroys microbial invaders, heals wounds and damages its own tissues. The acute phase of inflammation is characterized by microvascular changes, and activation of granulocytic cells. Cells from the monocytes lineage predominate in the mature or chronic inflammatory response.

Acute inflammation can move in several directions, toward chronic inflammation, the formation of an abscess, wound healing or resolution. As the inflammatory response gradually fades, resolution can occur. The autoimmune diseases are the consequence of long-lasting inflammation. Resolution is an active process that stops the collateral damage and moves back to homeostasis.

Exudate is not just pus, it is an organized response to inflammation, it is a rich source of the fatty acids needed for the biosynthesis of anti-inflammatory mediators formed through the oxidation of omega-3 fatty acids. They target macrophages, endothelial and dendritic cells to produce IL-10 and stimulate macrophage phagocytosis. Three types of modulators have been identified: lipoxins, resolvins and protectins. Resolvins E and D are biologically active in arthritis, asthma, *periodontitis*, dry eye, cardiovascular disease, inflammatory bowel disease and other inflammatory conditions. Resolvin E1 and D1 can attenuate pain more effectively than morphine. The mediators affect signaling in central and peripheral ganglia to reduce the perception of pain.

The most important plasma-derived mediators of inflammation are the products of complement activation, which provoke vasodilation, chemotaxis of granulocytes and the secretion of mediators from inflammatory cells. Complement is a system of enzymes and proteins that function in both the innate and adaptive branches of the immune system as soluble means of protection against pathogens. Complement can be activated in three ways: *via* the classical pathway, lectin pathway and alternative pathway. Functions of complement include lysis of bacteria, cells, and viruses; promotion of phagocytosis (opsonization), triggering inflammation and secretion of immunoregulatory molecules and clearance of immune complexes from circulation. Multiple inflammatory mediators (histamine, serotonin, prostaglandins, leukotrienes, superoxide anion and nitric oxide) released from activated cells provoke tissue injury. The inflammatory response involves a complex interaction between the nervous system and inflammatory cells.

Dysregulation of the immune response is a key element that underpins pathogenicity of multiple immune and inflammatory diseases. There are two broad categories of disease that reflect the two extremes of immune dysregulation. The first group is characterised by deficiencies of the immune system. The second group of diseases includes those in which there are features of an excessive, overactive or inappropriately persistent immune response. Autoimmune diseases are most likely caused by a response of the cells of the adaptive immune system (*i.e.*, T cells and B cells) to tissue of the host. So, in many autoimmune diseases auto-antibodies are found that can be more or less specific for a given disease. The cause of most of the autoimmune diseases is not known but they are likely to arise through multiple mechanisms.

In autoimmune diseases many autoantibodies are produced. Laboratory methods to detect particular autoantibodies have provided the clinician with valuable tools. Serology is of particular value in the early stage of disease when clinical signs and symptoms are often not complete, then the autoantibody profile can be diagnostic.

Autoantibodies are markers of chronic immune-inflammation and rheumatic diseases. Some of these are specific for one disease, while others can be found in several diseases.

Rheumatoid factors are autoantibodies to IgG molecules, being produced in many inflammatory conditions, but they are important for diagnosing rheumatoid arthritis (RA), Sjögren's syndrome (SS), hypergammaglobulinemic purpura and mixed cryoglobulinemia. Rheumatoid factor (RF) is directed to the Fc gamma-chains of IgG molecules. In clinical practice, laboratories tend to test only for IgM RF but RF can belong to all major immunoglobulin classes (IgG, IgA, IgM, IgD and IgE). All these classes of RF are produced locally in the rheumatoid synovial membrane. The most common methods for quantifying RF are ELISA or nephelometric assays.

Anti citrullinated peptide antibodies (ACPA) form a family of autoantibodies which includes antiperinuclear factor (APF), anti-keratin antibodies (AKA) and anti-Sa. ACPA is a single cyclic citrullinated peptide and has a 3-dimentional structure. Autoantibodies to citrullinated peptides have become more specific marker for RA. However, not only RA patients react to these proteins by producing significant amounts of ACPA. Patients with early undifferential arthritis, positive ACPA predicts later development of classic erosive RA. The sensitivity of the ACPA test is around 50% at the onset of RA and can rise up to 85% later in the development of the disease. It is common in RF-positive patients but can be found in around 25% of seronegative patients as well. ACPA can be detected by ELISA and immunoblotting methods using citrullinated proteins or peptides.

Antinuclear antibodies (ANA) are a diverse group of antibodies, often directed to large cellular complexes containing protein and nucleic acid components. The most frequently occurring ANA react with components of DNA-protein or RNA-protein complexes.

ANA can give important clues to diagnosis and prognosis, especially in patients suspected of, or suffering from systemic lupus erythematosus (SLE), Sjögren's syndrome (SS), progressive systemic sclerosis (scleroderma) (SSc), Raynaud's syndrome (RS), poly-/and dermatomyositis (PM/DM), mixed connective tissue disease (MCTD) and juvenile idiopathic arthritis (JIA).

Frequency of ANA in Autoimmune and Non-rheumatic Diseases (Autoimmune Disease and Sensitivity) are following:

Systemic lupus erythematosus	– 90-95%
Scleroderma	– 60-80%
Mixed connective tissue disease	– 100%
Polymyositis/dermatomyositis	– 60%

Contd.....

Rheumatoid arthritis	– 50%
Sjögren's syndrome	– 40-70%
Drug-induced lupus	– 90%
Juvenile chronic arthritis	– 70%
Hashimoto's thyroiditis	– 45%
Graves' disease	– 50%
Autoimmune hepatitis	– 50%
Primary pulmonary hypertension	– 40%

Clinical associations of autoantibodies in SLE.

Antigen specificity, clinical associations and sensitivity (%) are the following: dsDNA is the marker for active lupus, correlated with renal disease in 40-70%; Ro/SS-A in 40-60% and La/SS-B in 15% correlated with Sjögren syndrome. Sm occurring in 5-30% in lupus.

Antiphospholipid antibodies (aPL) (anticardiolipin antibodies (aCL) and lupus anticoagulant (LA)) target protein/lipid complexes of importance for coagulation processes. They predispose to thromboembolic events, thrombocytopenia and pregnancy loss. aPL are antibodies directed at certain serum protein complexes to phospholipid molecules. Presence of functionally procoagulant aPL can be screened for by finding an abnormally prolonged activated partial thromboplastin time (APTT). aPL were originally detected by false-positive tests for syphilis using the Wassermann reaction. Subsequently positive reactivity in the anticardiolipin ELISA assay and in the lupus anticoagulant test was shown to depend on binding of autoantibodies to a serum co-factor, which in the case of the anticardiolipin ELISA is $\beta 2$–glycoprotein I ($\beta 2$GPI) and in the lupus anticoagulant assay may be either $\beta 2$GPI or prothrombin.

Lupus anticoagulants do not function as anticoagulants but conversely as procoagulants. They block the assembly of the prothrombinase complex, giving rise to prolonged coagulation assays in vitro *e.g.* prolonged APTT, dilute Russell viper venom time or kaolin clotting time. LA is an inappropriate name for the procoagulant autoantibodies since they appear not only in SLE but in primary antiphospholipid syndrome (APS), defined as patients experiencing venous or arterial thrombotic events, recurrent fetal loss and thrombocytopenia.

Anticardiolipin antibodies (aCL) are detected by ELISA. The most important phospholipid binding protein attaching to the cardiolipin is $\beta 2$GPI, which acts as a co-factor in the test. Autoantibodies to $\beta 2$GPI and to cardiolipin/$\beta 2$GPI complex give rise to positive results of importance for diagnosing a procoagulant state. aCL transiently appear in several infections and permanently in syphilis. The antibodies may belong to all three major IgG classes but IgG aCL antibodies are those most closely related to procoagulant activity. Both aCL antibodies and LA can be found in many rheumatic diseases but most commonly in patients with SLE.

Antineutrophil cytoplasmic antibodies (ANCA) describes a number of circulating autoantibodies specifically directed against the cytoplasmic constituents of neutrophils and monocytes. Two ANCA patterns were originally identified by indirect immunofluorescence:

the cytoplasmic (c-ANCA) and the perinuclear (p-ANCA) patterns. The classical c-ANCA is associated with antibodies reacting with the 29-30 kDa elastinolytic enzyme, serine proteinase-3 (PR3). This is composed of 229 amino acids and found in the azurophilic granules of neutrophils and monocytes. The classical p-ANCA pattern is associated with antibodies to myeloperoxidase (MPO), a 140 kDa heterodymeric enzyme also associated with the antimicrobial properties of neutrophils. ANCA associated with primary small vessel systemic necrotizing vasculitis target lysosomal enzymes, first and foremost proteinase 3 and myeloperoxidase. ANCA are very strongly expressed in drug-induced syndromes, *e.g.* drug-induced lupus-like syndrome and drug-induced vasculitis. Proteinase 3-ANCA levels may reflect disease activity in granulomatosis with polyangiitis (GPA) but not always, whereas myeloperoxidase-ANCA levels do not show such associations.

Acute phase reactants that include a number of serum proteins (among them C-reactive protein [CRP] and fibrinogen) can reflect ongoing inflammation and be represented by an increased erythrocyte sedimentation rate [ESR]. Monitoring the levels of these proteins may be helpful in evaluating disease progression.

The acute phase response occurs in a wide variety of inflammatory conditions including various infections, trauma, malignancies, inflammatory rheumatic disorders and certain immune reactions to drugs.

The acute phase proteins are produced by hepatocytes after signals received from cytokines, *e.g.* interleukin 6, interleukin 1 and TNFα. These proteins will increase by about 25% during an inflammatory state but some *e.g.* CRP can increase more than a hundred times.

The most important acute phase proteins which increase during inflammation (positive reactants) are CRP, fibrinogen, α1-antitrypsin, haptoglobin, ceruloplasmin, serum amyloid protein A and several complement components, especially complement C3.

In chronic inflammation some proteins decrease in serum due to deficient hepatocyte production (negative reactants) and these include albumin, transthyretin and transferrin.

Currently the most popular markers of inflammation are CRP and ESR. While CRP concentrations increase and decrease very rapidly, ESR values change slowly, therefore ESR is an indirect measure of acute phase protein concentration.

CRP values of less than 0.1-0.2 mg/dl are considered as normal, those between 0.2 and 1 mg/dl can be seen without obvious signs of inflammation but values higher than 1.0 mg/dl should lead to a clinical manifestation.

Complement levels in plasma represent a balance between increased production during inflammation and consumption by circulating or tissue-deposited immune complexes.

CHAPTER 1

Rheumatoid Arthritis

Abstract: Rheumatoid arthritis (RA) is a chronic inflammatory disease which affects around 0.5-1% of the population. RA is characterized by symmetric, erosive arthritis of the synovial joints and with various extra-articular features. The progressive destruction of the articular cartilage leads to deformation and loss of function of affected joints. The primary affected area is synovium, at the site where the "pannus" is developed. RA is characterized by a poor outcome, but the course may be varied. RA that is not controlled is associated with a reduction in life expectancy. The risk of atherosclerosis and lymphoma development is increased in RA . The etiopathogenesis of RA is partially understood, as it is a multifactorial disease and is determined by genetic as well as environmental factors. Class II major histocompatibility genes are responsible for about 30% of genetic susceptibility to RA. The autoantibody profile can be diagnostic, specifically rheumatoid factor (RA) and antibodies to cyclic-cytrullinated peptides (ACPA) more specific marker. RA is an economical burden for patients and society. Substantial advances have been made in the management at RA. Currently, methotrexate is the basic conventional synthetic (cs) disease-modifying antirheumatic drugs (DMARD) in RA treatment. It may be used in combination with biologic drugs.

Following the introduction of the treatment recommendations for RA in 2016 by the EULAR, and the introduction of biological (b) DMARDs and targeted synthetic (ts) DMARDs in the management of RA, special consideration must be taken in the selection of therapy for patients who do not respond to standard treatment.

Keywords: Antibodies to cyclic-cytrullinated peptides (ACPA), Biological DMARDs, Disease-modifying antirheumatic drugs (DMARDs), Erosions, Erosive arthritis, Leflunomide, Methotrexate, Pannus, Rheumatoid arthritis, Rheumatoid factor (RA), Synovium, Targeted synthetic DMARDs.

INTRODUCTION

RA is a chronic inflammatory disease which affects around 0.5-1% of the population, the highest rate occurring in American-Indian populations showing between 5.3 to 6.8%, and the lowest occurrence has been shown in populations from South Africa, Nigeria and South-East Asia, with an occurrence rate of 0.2% to 0.3% [1]. RA is characterized by symmetric, erosive arthritis of the synovial joints and with various extra-articular features. Typical articular symptoms include pain, stiffness and swelling. The progressive destruction of the articular cartilage leads to deformation and loss of function of affected joints. The primary affected area is synovium, at the site where the "pannus" is developed.

RA is usually characterized by a poor outcome, but the course may be varied. RA that is not controlled is associated with a reduction in life expectancy, which in some studies may be up to 6-7 years [1]. The risk of atherosclerosis and lymphoma development is increased in RA [2].

RA is an economical burden for both patients and society, which is calculated in terms of direct and indirect costs. Direct costs are where actual payments are made, *e.g.* treatment and hospitalization costs, while indirect costs are those resulting from loss of resources, *e.g.* loss of productivity.

Substantial advances have been made in the field of rheumatology in the past 20 years, particularly in the management at RA. Following the introduction of the treatment recommendations for RA in 2016 by the European League Against Rheumatism (EULAR) [3], and the introduction of biological (b) disease-modifying antirheumatic drugs (DMARDs) and targeted synthetic (ts) DMARDs in the management of RA, special consideration must be taken in the selection of therapy for patients who do not respond to standard treatment.

ETIOPATHOGENESIS

The etiopathogenesis of RA is only partially understood, as it is a multifactorial disease and is determined by genetic as well as environmental factors [4]. 50-60% of the risk of developing RA is due to genetics [5, 6]. The familial RA occurrences are about 10-30% of patients, in 12-15% of monozygotic twins and in 3-4% of dizygotic twins [7]. Genes play an important role in the susceptibility to RA. Class II major histocompatibility genes are responsible for about 30% of genetic susceptibility to RA [8]. Susceptibility to RA and disease severity, is connected particularly with the human leukocyte antigen (HLA) located on the short arm of chromosome 6 (6p21.3) [8]. The most important genetic associations are class II major histocompatibility genes, especially those containing a specific 5 amino acid sequence in the hypervariable region of HLA-DR. The susceptibility to RA is associated with the third hypervariable region of DRβ-chains, from amino acids 70 through 74 amino acid sequence which consists of glutamine – leucine – arginine – alanine – alanine (QKRAA) and is called "shared epitope" [8]. This epitope is found in DR4, DR14 and some DR1β chains.

The first non-HLA genetic association with RA is the protein tyrosine phosphatase-22 (*PTPN22*) candidate gene, which encodes a lymphoid-specific protein tyrosine phosphatase, that downregulates T cell receptor signaling.

PTPN22 is a phosphatase that regulates the phosphorylation status of several kinases important to T cell activation [9].

The *PADI* (peptidylarguinine deiminase) genes are responsible for the post-translational modification of arginine to citrulline. An extended haplotype in the *PAD 4* gene provides the most promising coding for RA [10].

Many other genes that are connected with immune regulation are also connected with RA, which is a polygenic disease.

RA is triggered by environmental factors, enhanced by genetic predisposition in combination with altered immune responses. For example *Porphyromonas gingivalis,* during periodontal diseases and tobacco smoking [11], encourages anti-cylic citrullinated peptide antibodies (ACPAs) production which has a crucial role in RA pathogenesis. Smoking is an important and proven risk factor, as it is connected with increased production of autoantibodies, especially ACPA and RF and with increased occurrence of extraarticular symptoms [11]. The polycyclic aromatic hydrocarbons (PAHs) present in tobacco smoke activate the aryl hydrocarbon receptor (AHR), which being a transcription factor, binds to response elements of xenobiotic (XRE), which regulates the expression of multiple genes [11].

The genetic associations of the HLA shared epitope alleles in the development of RA indicates that the disease is partially driven by T cells [12], and especially with CD4+T cells, which are a dominant cells type (add up to 30-50% all cells type) in the synovium of RA patients [13]. This subpopulation of T cells is capable of suppressing immune response [13].

For the development of RA a decrease in immunological self-tolerance is required. Human naïve CD4+T cells, depending on the cytokine environment in which they are currently in, divide into distinct cell subset, such as Th1, Th2, Th17 cells, regulatory T cells (Treg) and T follicular helper cells [14]. Th1 cells function to activate macrophages in ways that enhance microbial killing. Th1 cells are characterized by the profile of cytokines they produce INFγ. Th2 cells function in responses against parasitic infestations, and secrete cytokines such as IL-4, IL-5 and IL-13. IL-4 induces the production of IgG4 and IgE. Th2 cells play key roles in atopic and allergic disease. Th17 cells participate in host defense against fungal infections and extracellular bacteria. Th 17 cells are typical pro-inflammatory cells that promote inflammatory responses in tissues and the development of autoimmune diseases.

Specific populations of CD4+ T cells (Tregs or CD4+CD25+) express regulatory functions. These cells are required to maintain homeostasis of the immune system by preventing the activation of self-reactive lymphoid populations. Treg cells are involved in the inhibition of activation of the immune system and maintain immune homeostasis and tolerance to self-antigens.

Th17 and Treg cell differentiation pathways are interconnected, meaning that balance between them is important for correct immune homeostasis [15].

Th 17 cells through the production of proinflammatory cytokines such as IL-17, IL-1β, IL-6, IL-21, IL-23, TNFα and GM-CSF are necessary for the induction and maintenance of autoimmune tissue inflammation and contribute to the differentiation and proliferation of osteoclasts, which cause bone resorption [16]. Th17 cells can also produce IL-21, which is a major regulator of IgG production and T-dependent humoral responses [17].

The function of Treg during a phase of homeostatic control may predict if an autoimmune disease will occur. However, in the chronic inflammatory phase the increased number of Treg cells may even be negative. They may cause inhibition of the immune response, contributing to a change in inflammatory processes, leading to chronic autoimmune inflammation. Treg cells inhibit immunologic responses in many ways, including cytotoxic factors, anti-inflammatory cytokines (*e.g.* IL-10, TGFβ, IL-35), metabolic disruption or by changing the maturation and function of antigen presenting cells [14]. In RA, patients' Treg cell count is higher in synovial fluid, comparing to peripheral blood, and there is still persistent inflammation in the joints. This means that these cells are not very effective in the control of inappropriate activation of the immune system [18]. Treg cells present in the RA synovial fluid may have an increased ability to suppress both T cell proliferation and production of proinflammatory cytokines (*e.g.* TNFα, INFγ), but disease is still able to progress [19]. This can be a result of interactions between Tregs and cytokines at the site of inflammation. Cytokines such as TNFα, IL-6, IL-15 and IL-1 present in the rheumatic joint are able to increase the number of infiltrating regulatory T cells and are able to impair their suppressive function [19]. The circulating Treg cells that can suppress proliferation of the effector T cells are unable to inhibit the proinflammatory cytokine secretion from activated T cells and monocytes [19]. Treg cells in the presence of pro-inflammatory cytokine-rich environment will change to pathogenic T cells [19].

Different extra – articular manifestations may be caused by abnormal systemic immune responses. The structure of the synovial vasculature is an ideal environment for innate and adaptive immune responses, making it one of the main targets in RA.

Macrophages and dendritic cells are the first line of defense in immunity, but pro-inflammatory stimuli can shift their whole metabolism toward glycolysis and away from oxidative phosphorylation. The altered metabolic pathways can drive cytokine production to produce damage in joints and other tissues. Succinate is critical in the inflammatory response in macrophages. It shifts macrophage metabolism toward glycolysis, which can drive IL-1 and other inflammatory cytokines. At the same time, succinate changes the function of mitochondria, which begin to produce reactive oxygen species that increase the production of IL-1β and other proinflammatory cytokines. The Krebs cycle, which most cells use to produce energy, is suddenly used to aid the production of inflammatory cytokines. It is a new way to look at cytokine dysregulation as a result of inflammatory changes. Developing research now looks at targets other than succinate. Many of the enzymes active in glycolysis are also recognized antigens commonly seen in rheumatoid disease. One of the key enzymes involved in glycolysis is enolase, known mainly as an autoantigen involved in rheumatoid arthritis.

Synovial cells are similar to a localized tumor that destroy articular cartilage, subchondral bone, tendons, and ligaments resulting in loss of articular cartilage and bone. Joint destruction is caused by synovial hyperplasia. The cells of the immune system (T, B cells, monocytes/macrophages, mastocytes, dendritic cells) as well as synovial cells (fibroblasts, endothelial cells, pericytes), chondrocytes, and bone cells (osteocytes, osteoblasts, osteoclasts) produce and release proinflammatory cytokines and matrix – degrading enzymes. Bone and cartilage destruction are mainly controlled by osteoclasts and fibroblasts – like synoviocytes, respectively.

Activation of synovial innate immunity causes increased vascular leakage into the synovium and it can produce chemoattractants that recruit immune cells to the joint. Dendritic cells than process the antigens. Antigen presentation can occur in the synovial germinal centers or in central lymphoid organs after the dendritic cells have processed the antigens and migrate *via* the lymphatics. Paracrine and autocrine pathways can lead to activation of fibroblast-like and macrophage-like synoviocytes in the synovial intimal lining. T helper type 1 (Th1) or Th17 cytokines can aid in increasing the network, and Th2 cytokines aid in suppressing it.

Environmental stresses can lead to post-transcriptional modification of proteins, specifically citrullination of arginine residues, in mucosal surfaces of the synovium. Patients with RA can develop antibodies against these modified proteins with production of RFs and ACPAs [20]. ACPA recognizes an antigen – citrulline. This non-standard amino acid is produced by the post-translational modification of arginine residues by the enzyme peptidylarginine deiminase. ACPA are present early in the course of RA, and can precede onset of symptoms by up to 10 years [20].

RA concerns peripheral joints, however immune disorders are not limited to the places where inflammation is induced but also are systemic. Mononuclear cells secrete pro- and anti-inflammatory cytokines in abnormal amounts. Proinflammatory cytokines involved in the pathogenesis of RA are TNFα, IL-1β, IL-6, IL-15 and IL-17, as well as matrix metalloproteinases. Pro-inflammatory (IL-1, IL-6, TNFα, IL-17) and anti-inflammatory (IL-10, TGFβ) cytokines and chemokines (chemotactic cytokines) provide molecular signals for communication between cells, and play significant roles in maintaining and regulating inflammatory reactions and cause disease perpetuation.

T and B lymphocytes, monocytes/macrophages, neutrophils, and mast cells contain surface receptors that bind to soluble factors, antigens, or other cellular components that cause activation of these cells. Activation of lymphocytes and cellular components of the inflammatory response triggers a cascade of intracellular biochemical events, called signal transduction.

Dysregulated extracellular mediators trigger abnormal intracellular signal transduction. Dysfunction of intracellular signal transduction effects cell activation, proliferation, migratory capacity and cell survival which all contribute to inflammation. One of the more important intracellular signal transduction pathways involved in the pathogenesis of RA include:

• Nuclear factor kappa B (NFkB),
• Mitogen associated protein kinases (MAPKs),
• Phosphoinositide 3 kinase (PI3K)/Akt,
• Signal transducers and activators of transcription (STATs).

The MAPK, spleen tyrosine kinase (Syk), NFkB and Janus-associated kinase (JAK), JAK/STAT intracellular signaling pathways are triggered by cytokines bound to their receptors. NFkB is expressed in the synovial tissue of RA patients [21]. It plays an important role in connecting intercellular signals by cytokine-mediated activation pathways. NFkB pathway is a major regulator of pro-inflammatory cytokine production and is activated by IL-1, TNFα and TLR signaling [21]. It is an important link between synovial inflammation, hyperplasia and matrix degradation, because it regulates receptor activator of nuclear factor kB (RANK) – an effector in joint destruction by mediating osteoclastogenesis [21].

There are additional kinase pathways identified, which include JAK, Syk, Bruton's tyrosine kinase (Btk), and PI3K pathways. The JAK/STAT pathways in RA play a key role [22]. The JAK/STAT pathway is activated by many cytokines, interferons and growth factors. The mediators of many cytokine signals are JAK due to receptors, that activate intracellular signaling pathways. Dysregulated

JAK1, JAK2, JAK3, and TYK2 signaling is associated with hematologic malignancies, autoimmune disorders, and immune deficient conditions [22]. Different cytokines use different JAKs. When specific cytokines bind to a cell surface receptor, JAKs associated with the intracellular portion of the receptor are activated and transmit signals to the nucleus to initiate gene transcription and production of cytokines and other immune mediators. Dysregulated expression of cytokines, and therefore overactivated JAK pathways signaling in RA, leads to chronic inflammation and tissue destruction [22].

Syk is an intracellular tyrosine kinase present in the synovium of patients with RA. It is an important modulator of immune signaling and is involved in the production of cytokines and metalloproteinases in RA patients. Bruton's tyrosine kinase is an important enzyme in the development, differentiation, and signaling of B-lymphocytes as well as mast cell activation. Btk is a critical part of the B-cell-receptor signaling pathway, which drives B-cell activation.

The synovial pannus is formed by rheumatoid arthritis synovial fibroblasts (RASFs), which are found in the synovium of joints, causing hyperplasia and multiple layers. Normal fibroblast-like synoviocytes (FLS) are mesenchymal-derivied cells that express extracellular mesenchymal-derived cells that express extracellular matrix (ECM) proteins such as vimentin, type IV and V collagens, and adhesion molecules such as integrins [23]. FLS produce UDP-glucose 6-dehydrogenase, an enzyme needed for the production of hyaluronic acid. FLS express cadherin-11, a selective adhesion molecule, which is essential for maintaining the integrity of the normal synovium [25]. Cadherin-11 also regulates the secretion of IL-6. Chronic inflammation induces FLS modifications, giving rise to the RASF phenotype and the formation of synovial pannus. Activated fibroblasts act like tumor cells, they are resistant to apoptosis, are able to survive in extreme conditions, have increased migration, reduced contact inhibition, reduced attachment-dependent growth, and an ability to invade and even to "metastatise" [24]. RASFs destroy cartilage and they are able to migrate out of the synovial tissue to distant cartilage through the vascular system, aiding in the spread of the disease to healthy cartilage of distant joints [26]. Microbial components or endogenous ligands such as RNA derived from necrotic cells might activate RASFs *via* TLR signalling and thus induce the expression of pro-inflammatory cytokines and chemokines. The increase of pro-inflammatory molecules results in the attraction and accumulation of immune cells in the synovium, causing a chronic inflammatory response [24].

Inflammatory cytokines IL-1β and TNFα, produced by macrophage-like cells that line the synovium, stimulate the production of IL-6. These cytokines also stimulate the production of matrix-degrading enzymes by RASFs, such as matrix metalloproteinases (MMPs) and IL-15, which induces the the production of TNFα and IL-17 by T-cells, which in turn stimulate the expression of IL-15 and IL-6 by RASFs [24].

Adipokines such as adiponectin, visfatin, resistin, leptin, chimerin and omentin are produced by adipose tissue in joints, as well as RASFs and are associated with disease severity [24]. This suggests a role in the pathogenesis of RA. Adipokines can contribute to the progression of inflammation and matrix degradation in RA [25]. Many adipokines are increased in the synovium, the synovial fluid and/or the serum of RA patients compared to OA patients [25].

The main mediators of tissue destruction in joints are MMPs (collagenases, gelatinases, stromelysins, matrilysins, membrane-type MMPs and adamalysisns). MMPs regulate many biological processes, including transcription, proenzyme activation, and inhibition by natural inhibitors. The expression of MMPs is regulated by tissue inhibitors of metalloproteinases (TIMPs). Cathepsins B, K and L are involved in the degradation of bone and cartilage. The high level of MMP-3 suggests an important role in the progression of erosions of the cartilage. Plasmin, uPA and tPA also contribute to tissue destruction in RA.

The role of osteoclasts in bone destruction in RA is very important. RA patients develop local bone erosion and destruction of affected joints containing synovial membrane, and also suffer from generalized osteoporosis *via* systemic inflammation. Osteoclast-free mice are protected from bone erosion in several mouse RA models [26].

Osteoclasts are multinucleated cells of haematopoietic origin, which are formed from mononuclear precursors by cell fusion that is regulated by two factors: macrophage colony-stimulating factor (M-CSF) and the RANK/RANKL (receptor activator of nuclear factor ligand) couple. At the site of bone erosion in RA, osteoclasts may derive from peripheral blood mononuclear cells, synovial mononuclear cells, subchondral bone cells and from monocyte progenitors that infiltrate the synovial membrane.

Synovial fibroblast, osteoclasts and chondrocytes express cathepsins, collagenases and a vacuolar-type adenosine triphosphatase (ATPase) which could contribute to bone matrix degradation. Proinflammatory cytokines like as TNFα, IL-1β, IL-6, IL-15 and IL-17 are able to activate cells capable of producing matrix-degrading enzymes.

The rheumatoid pannus contains mononuclear cells exhibiting tartate-resistant acid phosphatase (TRAP) activity, a specific marker of osteoclasts.

The result of chronic inflammation is the accumulation of osteoclast precursors, specifically mononuclear cells. Many cytokines are involved in osteoclastogenesis such as TNFα, IL-1β, IL-6 or M-CSF in inflamed joints. Activated RASFs are the source for RANKL, activating RANK bearing osteoclast precursor cells.

Interaction between ACPA and citrullinated vimentin, expressed on the surface of the monocyte/ macrophage cells, stimulates their differentiation into osteoclasts and therefore promotes bone loss [27].

Cartilage destruction in RA may be due to the production of matrix-degrading enzymes and their inhibitors by activated RASFs and by the deregulation of chondrocyte function through the release of cytokines and other mediators from the synovium.

RA predominates in women, the female to–male ratio is between 2: 1 and 3: 1. Female predominance suggests that sex hormones and reproductive factors influence both RA development and severity. Pregnancy often induces remission of the disease in the last trimester. More than three quarters of pregnant patients with RA improve in the first or second trimester, but 90% of these experience a recurrence of disease activity, associated with a rise in RF titers in the weeks or months after delivery. The mechanism of protection is not fully understood but may be due to the expression of suppressive cytokines such as IL-10 during pregnancy [28].

RA is a autoimmune disease, however a main arthritogenic autoantigen has not been found yet. RF is not specific to RA, nor has it always been present in the disease. This has lead to doubts about its role in the pathogenesis. Circulating IgM-RF is commonly seen in healthy individuals following immunization, particularly the elderly, or those with chronic infection without any sign of joint disease. RFs, present mostly as IgM-RF, but detectable also as IgG-RF and IgA-RF in some subgroups of patients, are thought to form immune complexes activating complement in the joint. This leads to increased vascular permeability and the release of chemotactic factors recruiting immune effectors cells to the joints.

ASSESSMENT

Laboratory methods to detect autoantibodies are important tools used in clinical practice. Serology is valuable in the early stages of RA, when clinical signs and symptoms are often not complete. This autoantibody profile can be diagnostic, specifically rheumatoid factor (RA) and antibodies to cyclic-cytrullinated peptides (ACPA), which have become a more specific marker for RA [29].

Rheumatoid factors are autoantibodies to IgG molecules, being produced in many inflammatory conditions, but they are important for diagnosing rheumatoid arthritis (RA), Sjögren's syndrome (SS), hypergammaglobulinemic purpura and mixed cryoglobulinemia. Rheumatoid factor (RF) is directed to the Fc gamma-chains of IgG molecules. In clinical practice, laboratories tend to test only for IgM RF but RF can belong to all major immunoglobulin classes (IgG, IgA, IgM, IgD and IgE). All these classes of RF are produced locally in the rheumatoid synovial membrane. The most common methods for quantifying RF are ELISA or nephelometric assays.

Anti citrullinated peptide antibodies (ACPA) form a family of autoantibodies which includes antiperinuclear factor (APF), anti-keratin antibodies (AKA) and anti-Sa. ACPA is a single cyclic citrullinated peptide and has a 3-dimentional structure. Antibodies to citrullinated peptides have become more specific marker for RA. However, not only RA patients react to these proteins by producing significant amounts of ACPA. Patients with early undifferential arthritis, positive ACPA predicts later development of classic erosive RA. The sensitivity of the ACPA test is around 50% at the onset of RA and can rise up to 85% later in the development of the disease [29]. It is common in RF-positive patients but can be found in around 25% of seronegative patients as well. ACPA can be detected by ELISA and immunoblotting methods using citrullinated proteins or peptides.

Currently the most widely used markers of inflammation are CRP and ESR in RA.

Imaging Procedures

Ultrasonography may be helpful at early stages of the disease to show synovitis of involved joints as well as to detect erosions of smaller joints.

Conventional radiographic examinations are the gold standard for diagnosing joint damage, but the absence of erosions on X-rays does not exclude RA. Radiographic examinations of the hands, wrist and feet are important to monitor disease progression. Scoring systems have been developed to assess the extent and changes of damage seen of X-ray images, such as the modified Sharp-van der Heijde score [30].

Magnetic Resonance Imaging (MRI) of wrist and finger joints is an important method for early diagnosis of RA. Synovitis and bone marrow edema may be found. MRI shows erosions earlier than with X-rays, however due to high costs it has not been used yet in every day clinical practice.

Classification Criteria

The Classification Criteria for RA (1987 ACR) [31] are:

1. Morning stiffness
2. Arthritis of at least three areas
3. Arthritis of hand joints
4. Symmetrical arthritis
5. Rheumatoid nodules
6. Serum rheumatoid factor
7. Radiographic changes (erosions or juxta-articular osteoporosis).

A diagnosis can be placed if 4 or more criteria are met.

The Classification Criteria for RA (2010 ACR and EULAR) [32] are:

A. Joint Involvement

1 big joint 0 points
2-10 big joints 1 point
1-3 small joints 2 points
4-10 small joints 3 points
>10 joints 5 points

B. Serology

RF and ACPA negative 0 points
RF or ACPA in low titer 2 points
RF or ACPA in high titer 3 points

C. Acute Phase Indicators

CRP and ESR normal 0 points
Elevated CRP or raised ESR 1 point

D. Duration of symptoms

<6 weeks 0 points
≥6 weeks 1 point
≥6 points diagnosis of RA confirmed.

Patients must meet two mandatory requirements for the classification criteria to be applied. Firstly, there must be clinical evidence of synovitis (*i.e.* swelling) in at least one joint. All joints of a full joint count may be assessed for this purpose with the exception of the DIP joints, the first MTP joint, and the first carpometacarpal joint as these joints are typically involved in osteoarthritis. Secondly, the synovitis should not be due to another disease – for example, SLE, psoriatic arthritis and gout. RA is then diagnosed and classified according to the score where a total score of ≥6 (out of 10) is calculated from individual scores in four domains. These are (A) number and site of involved joints (score range 0-5); (B) serological abnormality (score range 0-3); (C) raised acute phase response (score range 0-1) and (D) symptom duration (score range 0-1). Patients with typical RA-type erosions seen on X-ray, with a typical history of RA may also be classified using the above criteria however the scoring system doesn't have to be applied in such cases [32].

DIAGNOSIS

During the early stages, the disease process can be altered or even reversed, therefore treatment during this period may have a much greater effect in slowing disease progression and achieving remission than treatment at a later stage. Early disease is defined as a period limited to weeks or months since the onset of disease. RF and ACPA have been detected in patients with RA years before the onset of symptoms, showing that the disease process begins before the onset of symptoms.

After diagnosis of RA, it is important to determine which patients are at risk of developing persistent and/or erosive arthritis. This prognostic assessment is important for optimizing treatment strategies. Female gender, cigarette smoking, duration of symptoms, the number of tender and swollen joints, hand involvement, the level of acute phase response, presence of RF and ACPA, and fulfillment of the 2010 ACR/EULAR diagnostic criteria for RA are all factors associated with disease progression. Treatment of early RA is started. The most important prognostic factors of radiological damage are a high acute phase response, the presence and titer of RA and ACPA at the beginning of the disease and early erosions at disease onset. In certain cases of RA, disease may progress rapidly. Identification of patients with rapid disease progression is very important.

Rapid progress of disease includes polyarthritis, extra-articular features (rheumatoid nodules, Sjögren syndrome, keratitis, pericarditis, diffuse interstitial pulmonary fibrosis, vasculitis and Felty's syndrome), high concentration of RF in serum, presence of immunologic complexes and genetic predisposition HLA – DR 1 0401, 0404, 0405, HLA-DR4 and smoking.

It is important to identify the main prognostic factors, which allows accurate prediction of disease progression. Aggressive treatment should be offered to patients with rapid progression of the disease. In 60% of patients with early RA, irreversible changes are visible during the first two years from disease onset.

Early therapy reduces the progress of radiological changes. The complete assessment of patients with RA not only includes determination of disease activity but also the effect of joint function. One out of four non treated RA patients requires alloplastic big joint replacement. After 5 years of disease 50% of RA patients are no longer able to work and after 10 years 100%, but after 20 years of disease over 80% of patients are permanently disabled.

Clinical types of RA are: slow progression in 35-60%, rapid progression in 60-90%, mild "selflimiting" in 5-10% and rapid onset in 10-25% and gradual in 50% of patients.

RA Progression: arthritis, joint damage, functional impairment, systemic changes and lastly disability and preterm death. Patients live on average 7 years shorter compared to the general population.

CLINICAL PICTURE

Typical articular signs and symptoms are pain, stiffness and swelling. Tenosynovitis, bursitis and carpal tunnel syndrome may be present. Because RA is a systemic disease, generalized weakness, weight loss or low grade fever and some extra-articular features such as sicca syndrome, nodules, and interstitial lung fibrosis may be observed.

The typical joint involvement at disease onset is swelling of the proximal interphalangeal (PIP) joints, the metarsophalangeal (MTP) joints and the wrist. The disease may also begin with involvement of one or a few joints and over time develop from undifferential oligo- or polyarthritis into a polyarticular, and symmetrical, disease. Sometimes the disease also starts with monoarthritis, for example, of the knee. Involvement of shoulders and hips at disease onset is rare. The typical clinical findings of inflamed joints are soft tissue swelling and tenderness, and limited motion. Detection of synovitis is essential for the diagnosis.

The deformities of joints are a consequence of chronic inflammation and radiographic damage. Involvement of the DIP joint is rare and should differentiate concurrent osteoarthritis, psoriatic arthritis or gout. Boutonniere deformity is typical in RA and is described as finger flexion of the PIP joint and hyperextension of the DIP joint. This is due to relaxation and volar displacement of the central tendon slip at the PIP joint. "Z-shaped" deformity of the thumb is similar with deformity due to flexion of the MCP joint and hyperextension of the IP joint at 90 degrees. A swan-neck deformity of the finger is another typical deformity for RA. This involves hyperextension of the PIP joint and flexion of the DIP joint. Deformities of the MCP joints include subluxation, ulnar drift and flexion deformities.

Potentially life-threatening involvement of the cervical spine is rare. The cause of inflammation is a presence of synovial articulation between the transverse ligaments of the atlas against the posterior aspect of the odontoid (dens). The transverse ligament acts as a belt and maintains odontoid process contact against the posterior surface of the atlas, preventing forward movement of C1 on C2. Synovitis of this joint causes erosions of the dens, compromising the transverse ligament and resulting in instability. The space between the anterior aspect of the odontoid process (C2) and the posterior surface of the anterior arch of the atlas (C1) measures ≤3 mm. If this space exceeds 5 mm the condition is defined as atlantoaxial (or C1-C2) subluxation. The consequence of synovitis in this area may be subluxation with neurological symptoms due to cervical myelopathy.

The elbow joint is frequently involved in RA. Loss of extension, supination and reduced flexion is observed. Shoulder involvement in RA, seen as synovitis leads to erosion and damage of the humeral head and glenoid fossa. The long head of the biceps muscle may rupture. The rotator cuff can also be involved with inflammation and destruction.

The hip is rarely involved in RA as opposed to knee involvement. Synovitis in the knee is a typical sign, followed by a loss of full knee extension and sometimes resulting in a Baker's cyst in the popliteal region. Rupture of this cyst produce general swelling of the calf and a clinical picture similar to that of deep vein thrombosis. Destruction of the knee joint leads to instability. This is due to laxity of the collateral and cruciate ligaments in women with physiological valgus.

The subtalar and mid-tarsal joints are more frequently involved than the ankle joint and sometimes we may observe subtalar dislocation. Forefoot deformity begins with synovitis of the MTP joints and involvement of the flexor tendons, which can result in clawing of the toes and dorsal dislocation of the MTP joints. The temporal mandibular joints are sometimes involved, accompanied by tenderness and painful limitation in mouth opening. Subcutaneous nodules form over pressure locations such as the proximal ulna, the occiput, palms of the hands, and Achilles tendons.

Because of the systemic and chronic nature of the disease, RA patients are at risk of developing extra-articular manifestations such as subcutaneous nodules, vasculitis, pericarditis, pulmonary nodules or interstitial fibrosis, mononeuritis multiplex, episcleritis or scleritis, and comorbidities including osteoporosis, premature atherosclerosis, muscle weakness, infections, and cancer.

In RA it has been observed that there is an increased generalized bone loss with increased occurrence of fractures. There is an increase in the occurrence of osteoporosis in RA patients. Osteoporosis is due to inflammation (*e.g.* cytokine release with osteoclast activation), and use of glucocorticoids and immobility. Muscle weakness and atrophy is due to neuropathy, use of steroids, and joint involvement. Secondary Sjögren's syndrome is a manifestation of RA with sicca symptoms from eyes and dryness of the mouth. There is an increased risk of malignancy in RA patients, especially lymphoma [2]. Vasculitis may lead to cutaneous ulceration or peripheral neuropathy (a mild distal sensory neuropathy and a severe sensory motor neuropathy – mononeuritis multiplex) or involvement of internal organs.

The kidney is rarely involved in RA but may be due to secondary amyloidosis (amyloidosis AA). It is a life threatening clinical extra – articular complication of RA. The most common symptoms are proteinuria, erythrocyturia, abdominal pain and chronic diarrhea. Effective anti-inflammatory therapy of RA and eradication of coexisting infections is the best way to decrease the risk of development and prevent progression of secondary amyloidosis.

Lung diseases associated with RA are pleuritis, interstitial pneumonitis and fibrosis and nodular lung disease. Pulmonary hypertension is rare.

Cardiac complications like pericarditis, myocarditis and endocardial inflammation may be present. Conduction defects are uncommon. Patients with RA have an increased risk of clinical coronary heart disease compared with age- and sex-matched non-RA patients, as atherosclerosis is correlated to the level of systemic inflammatory activity over time and the inflammatory process impacts on cardiovascular morbidity and mortality and accelerated coronary and extra-coronary atherosclerosis. Wislowska *et al.* [33] in a detailed study of rheumatoid patients using echocardiography, Holter monitors, and electrocardiography, was reported that 70% of patients with nodular disease and 40% of those with non-nodular RA have some cardiac involvement, including valve thickening or incompetence. Midtbo *et al.* [34] concluded that active RA is associated with lower LV systolic myocardial function despite normal ejection fraction and independent of traditional cardiovascular risk factors.

DISEASE ASSESSMENT

Disease evaluation before and after treatment includes: number of tender joints, number of swollen joints, pain in VAS scale, ESR, CRP, DAS28, SDAI, CDAI, duration of morning stiffness and disability degree HAQ [35], SF-36 [36].

Disease Assessment: SDAI, CDAI, DAS28

SDAI (The Simplified Disease Activity Index) [37] uses a sum of five untransformed, not weighted variables, including 28-SJC and 28-TJC, patient and investigator global assessment of disease activity on a VAS and CRP. Threshold definitions for remission, low, and moderate levels of disease activity are 3.3, 11, and 26, respectively.

CDAI (Clinical Disease Activity Index) [37] is a modification of SDAI without laboratory evaluation (CRP) to allow easy and fast clinical assessment. Thresholds for separating remission, low, and moderate levels of disease activity are 2.8, 10 and 22.

DAS28 (Disease Activity Score 28) **[38, 39]**

We measure the number of tender and swollen joints within 28:

Shoulder (2), elbow (2), knee (2), wrists (2), MCP (10) and PIP (10).

To calculate DAS 28 four variables are needed:

Joint pain/tenderness (0-28 joints)

Joint swelling (0-28 joints)

ESR 1-200 mm/h

Patient's global assessment of disease activity based on a visual analogue scale (VAS) 1-100 mm

0 – means no symptoms on this scale but 100 means unbearable.

Disease Activity Index Interpretation

DAS 28≥5.1 high activity

DAS 28 3.2-5.1 medium activity

DAS 28 2.6-3.2 small activity

DAS 28<2.6 remission.

Response to Treatment

DAS reduction by 1.2 or more – good response

DAS reduction 0.6-1.2 – medium response

DAS reduction below 0.6 – no response.

DAS 28 describes a 28-joint count and provides as much information as needed and correlates just as well as other measures, involving a more detailing count. DAS28 measures strictly correlate with disability and progression of radiological changes.

Functional disability is most commonly measured by the Stanford HAQ [40]. The shortened version, the Modified Health Assessment Questionnaire (MHAQ), reduces the number of criteria from 20 to 8, one for each of the eight components, and does not allow upgrading of scores by the use of technical devices or help by another person.

Remission Criteria ACR are: morning stiffness less than 15 minutes, without fatigue, without painful joints, without joint tenderness or pain in motion, without periarticular swelling, ESR<30 mm/h in women and ESR<20 mm/h in men [41, 42].

TREATMENT

Early diagnosis, early treatment and frequently monitoring of RA patients is important because of positive results in future outcomes. Precise control of disease activity in early stages of the disease is important to induce remission or to achieve a low disease activity and to prevent future damage and disability. The "treat to target" approach represents a treatment strategy which equals the disease activity of RA patients with low disease activity or remission. The patient is assessed every 1-3 months during active disease and treatment is changed until remission is achieved [43]. This "treat to target" is supported by the TICORA study [44] in which patients who underwent strict control of disease activity had less radiographic changes compared to patients treated with a standard treatment.

Disease-modifying antirheumatic drugs (DMARDs) are the group of drugs with different biochemical and pharmacokinetic way of action, which has a positive impact on radiological outcomes of joint damage (erosions and joint space narrowing).

Currently METHOTREXATE (MTX) is the basic conventional synthetic (cs) DMARD in RA treatment. It may be used in combination with biologic drugs. MTX is well absorb both orally and parenteral and quickly and widely distributed into tissues.

MTX leads to an increase of adenosine, which has a strong anti-inflammatory effect. MTX is a cytostatic antimetabolic drug, inhibiting the biosynthesis of nucleic acids' production. It causes the induction of p35 and stops the cell cycle in S phase. The mechanism of MTX involves its' resemblance to folic acid, that is important in monocarbonic groups transfer necessary for nucleotide biosynthesis. MTX resembles folic acid and is a competitive inhibitor of folate-dependent enzymes, such as dihydrofolate reductase (DHFR). These enzymes are involved in the pyrimidine (DNA) synthesis and *de novo* purine synthesis of DNA and RNA. DHFR inhibition by MTX leads to depletion of tetrahydrofolates that are essential for DNA, RNA and protein synthesis [45].

Initial dose of MTX is 10-15 mg/week, increased slowly to 25 mg/week. Side effects are: bone marrow toxicity, liver toxicity, interstitial pneumonitis and bronchiolitis, nauseous and mucous-membrane ulceration (GI side effects), interaction with alcohol and hair loss. Remission EULAR (DAS28<2.6) in 24 weeks of treatment occurred in 24% of patients treated with MTX orally and 34% of patients treated subcutaneously [46]. ACR20 response in 24 weeks occurred in 67% of patients treated orally with MTX and in 78% of patients treated subcutaneously [46]. MTX toxicities due to folate antagonism are: anemia, neutropenia, aphthosis, gastric ulcers. Other MTX toxicities are: rheumatoid nodule development, hepatic cirrhosis, somnolence and renal insufficiency. Control blood tests must be performed after 4 weeks and then after 8 weeks: morphology with platelets, liver function tests (AspAT, AlAT), prothrombin time and creatinine. For patients unable to tolerate oral MTX, subcutaneous or intramuscular injection may be administered once per week to limit some GI side effects. Alternatively folic acid may be used to decrease some adverse effects.

Other csDMARDs are leflunomide and sulfasalazine.

Leflunomide is an isoxazole derivative and a prodrug whose active metabolite is malononitrilamide A77 1726. It inhibits *de novo* pyrimidine synthesis, resulting in diverse antiproliferative and anti-inflammatory effects such as suppression of TNF-induced cellular responses and inhibition of matrix metalloproteinases and osteoclasts [47]. Leflunomide may increase the risk of fetal death and have teratogenic effects and should only be started if pregnancy is excluded and is not planned. Because of long half-life of leflunomide, a course of cholestyramine (3×8g daily for 11 days) can be given to aid clearance of the active compound. Without washout, elimination of leflunomide may take 2 years. Leflunomide stops proliferation of T lymphocytes and synthesis of pirymidin. Treatment is 10-20 mg/24 h.

Sulfasalazine (SSZ) is a 5-aminosalicylic acid derivative which is metabolized *via* the colonic intestinal flora to sulfapyridine and 5-aminosalicylic acid (5-ASA).

After absorption it is metabolized. Sulfapyridine is the active metabolite in RA, although its mechanism of action is unknown. SSZ is a DMARD used in the treatment of RA because of its good risk/benefit ratio.

Glucocorticoids (GCS) have anti-inflammatory and immunosuppressive effects. Short-term GCS should be started when initiating or changing csDMARDs in different dose and routes of administration, but should be tapered as rapidly as clinically possible. GCS treatment adverse effects include osteoporosis, hyperglycaemia, hypertension, skin fragility, peptic ulcer disease, premature atherosclerosis, cataracts, myopathy, osteonecrosis, infection, mood changes, sleep disturbances and weight gain. GCS therapy is a "bridging treatment" and should be stopped as soon as disease activity is controlled.

Biologic agents that target inflammatory cytokines and cells within the synovium and immune system are now used. Cytokine-blocking agents targeting TNF, interleukin-6, rituximab (B cell depleting antibodies) and costimulation blocking agents are used in RA after positive results in randomized, double-blind, placebo-controlled clinical trials (ATTRACT [48] and BeSt [49] with infliximab, COMET [50] and TEMPO [51] with etanercept, ARMADA [52] and PREMIER [53] with adalimumab, GO-BEFORE [54], GO-FORWARD [55] and GO-AFTER [56] with golimumab, RAPID1 [57] and RAPID2 [57] with certolizumab, AMBITION [58] with tocilizumab, DANCER [59] with rituximab) and trial with abatacept [60].

Infliximab is a human murine chimeric antibody against TNF. Adalimumab and golimumab are human monoclonal antibodies against TNF. Certolizumab pegol is a humanized antibody, in which the recombinant Fab' fragment that recognizes TNF has been conjugated with a polyethylene glycol chain. The PEGylation of the Fab' fragment increases its half-life and can also reduce its immunogenicity.

Etanercept is a TNF receptor fused to a human Fc molecule creating a bivalent TNF binding agent.

Adverse effects after TNFα blockade are severe infections (tuberculosis and others), demyelinisation syndrome, lymphoproliferative syndromes and antibodies (ANA, dsDNA, HACA) production.

Tocilizumab is the humanized monoclonal antibody that inhibits IL-6 receptor signaling through both its membrane bound and soluble forms.

Rituximab is a chimeric monoclonal antibody containing humanized and murine sequences in its protein structure. On binding to cells expressing CD20, rituximab induces cell death through a variety of mechanisms that include complement-mediated lysis, antibody-dependent cellular killing and apoptosis induction.

Abatacept is a soluble recombinant fully human protein that comprises the extracellular domain of CTLA4 and the Fc portion of an IgG1 molecule that has been modified to prevent complement activation. The T cell therefore receives one signal which tends to switch off the cell – the so-called "anergy" response.

Signal transduction proteins, such as kinases, have emerged as potential targets to modulate the immune system in RA. The effect of their activation results in translational or post-translational regulation of gene expression. They modulate the JAK signaling pathway and lead to the downstream inhibition of an interleukin and cytokine cascade [61].

Protein kinase inhibitors like tofacitinib and baricitinib are effective oral agents for the treatment of RA. Protein kinase inhibitors increases lipids, elevates liver enzymes, causes neutropenia and anemia, slightly increases creatinine levels, and have some gastrointestinal problems associated with it, all of which are manageable.

EULAR recommendations for the management of rheumatoid arthritis with synthetic and biological disease-modifying antirheumatic drugs: 2016 update [3].

Overarching Principles

A. Treatment of patients with RA should aim at the best care and must be based on a shared decision between the patient and the rheumatologist.
B. Treatment decisions are based on disease activity and other patient factors, such as progression of structural damage, comorbidities and safety issues.
C. Rheumatologists are the specialists who should primarily care for RA patients.
D. RA incurs high individual, medical and societal costs, all of which should be considered in its management by the treating rheumatologist.

Recommendations

1. Therapy with DMARDs should be started as soon as the diagnosis of RA is made.
2. Treatment should be aimed at reaching a target of sustained remission or low disease activity in every patient.
3. Monitoring should be frequent in active disease (every 1-3 months); if there is no improvement by at most 3 months after the start of treatment or the target has not been reached by 6 months, therapy should be adjusted.
4. MTX should be part of the first treatment strategy.
5. In patients with a contraindications to MTX (or early intolerance), leflunomide or sulfasalazine should be considered as part of the (first) treatment strategy.

6. Short-term glucocorticoids should be considered when initiating or changing csDMARDs in different dose regiments and routes of administration, but should be tapered as rapidly as clinically feasible.

7. If the treatment target is not achieved with the first csDMARD strategy, in the absence of poor prognostic factors, other csDMARD should be considered.

8. If the treatment target is not achieved with the first csDMARD strategy, when poor prognostic factors are present addition of a bDMARD or a tsDMARD (tofacitinib, baricitinib) should be considered; current practice would be to a start a bDMERD.

9. bDMARD and tsDMARDs should be combined with a csDMARD; in patients who cannot use csDMARDs as comedication, IL-6 pathway inhibitors and tsDMARDs may have some advantages compared with other bDMARDs.

10. If a bDMARD or tsDMARD has failed, treatment with another bDMARD or a tsDMARD should be considered, if one TNF inhibitor therapy has failed, patients may receive another TNF-inhibitor or an agent with another mode of action.

11. If a patient is in persistent remission after having tapered glucocorticoids, one can consider tapering bDMARDs, especially if this treatment is combined with a csDMARD.

12. If a patient is in persistent remission, tapering the csDMARD could be considered.

Tapering is seen as either dose reduction or prolongation of intervals between applications.

REFERENCES

[1]   Sangha O. Epidemiology of rheumatic diseases. Rheumatology (Oxford) 2000; 39 (Suppl. 2): 3-12.
      [http://dx.doi.org/10.1093/rheumatology/39.suppl_2.3] [PMID: 11276800]

[2]   Baecklund E, Iliadou A, Askling J, *et al.* Association of chronic inflammation, not its treatment, with increased lymphoma risk in rheumatoid arthritis. Arthritis Rheum 2006; 54(3): 692-701.
      [http://dx.doi.org/10.1002/art.21675] [PMID: 16508929]

[3]   Smolen JS, Landewé R, Bijlsma J, *et al.* EULAR recommendations for the management of rheumatoid arthritis with synthetic and biological disease-modifying antirheumatic drugs: 2016 update. Ann Rheum Dis 2017; 76(6): 960-77.
      [http://dx.doi.org/10.1136/annrheumdis-2016-210715] [PMID: 28264816]

[4]   Silman AJ, Pearson JE. Epidemiology and genetics of rheumatoid arthritis. Arthritis Res 2002; 4 (Suppl. 3): S265-72.
      [http://dx.doi.org/10.1186/ar578] [PMID: 12110146]

[5]   Bax M, van Heemst J, Huizinga TW, Toes RE. Genetics of rheumatoid arthritis: what have we learned? Immunogenetics 2011; 63(8): 459-66.
      [http://dx.doi.org/10.1007/s00251-011-0528-6] [PMID: 21556860]

[6]   Viatte S, Plant D, Raychaudhuri S. Genetics and epigenetics of rheumatoid arthritis. Nat Rev Rheumatol 2013; 9(3): 141-53.
      [http://dx.doi.org/10.1038/nrrheum.2012.237] [PMID: 23381558]

[7]   Reveille JD. Genetics studies in the rheumatic disease: present status and implications for the future. J Rheumatol 2005; 32 (Suppl. 72): 10-3.

[8]   Gregersen PK, Silver J, Winchester RJ. The shared epitope hypothesis. An approach to understanding the molecular genetics of susceptibility to rheumatoid arthritis. Arthritis Rheum 1987; 30(11): 1205-13.
[http://dx.doi.org/10.1002/art.1780301102] [PMID: 2446635]

[9]   Begovich AB, Carlton VE, Honigberg LA, *et al.* A missense single-nucleotide polymorphism in a gene encoding a protein tyrosine phosphatase (PTPN22) is associated with rheumatoid arthritis. Am J Hum Genet 2004; 75(2): 330-7.
[http://dx.doi.org/10.1086/422827] [PMID: 15208781]

[10]   Suzuki A, Yamada R, Chang X, *et al.* Functional haplotypes of PADI4, encoding citrullinating enzyme peptidylarginine deiminase 4, are associated with rheumatoid arthritis. Nat Genet 2003; 34(4): 395-402.
[http://dx.doi.org/10.1038/ng1206] [PMID: 12833157]

[11]   Källberg H, Ding B, Padyukov L, *et al.* Smoking is a major preventable risk factor for rheumatoid arthritis: estimations of risks after various exposures to cigarette smoke. Ann Rheum Dis 2011; 70(3): 508-11.
[http://dx.doi.org/10.1136/ard.2009.120899] [PMID: 21149499]

[12]   Andersson AK, Li C, Brennan FM. Recent developments in the immunobiology of rheumatoid arthritis. Arthritis Res Ther 2008; 10(2): 204-9.
[http://dx.doi.org/10.1186/ar2370] [PMID: 18373887]

[13]   Boissier MC, Assier E, Biton J, Denys A, Falgarone G, Bessis N. Regulatory T cells (Treg) in rheumatoid arthritis. Joint Bone Spine 2009; 76(1): 10-4.
[http://dx.doi.org/10.1016/j.jbspin.2008.08.002] [PMID: 19028128]

[14]   Noack M, Miossec P. Th17 and regulatory T cell balance in autoimmune and inflammatory diseases. Autoimmun Rev 2014; 13(6): 668-77.
[http://dx.doi.org/10.1016/j.autrev.2013.12.004] [PMID: 24418308]

[15]   Alunno A, Manetti M, Caterbi S, *et al.* Altered immunoregulation in rheumatoid arthritis: the role of regulatory T cells and proinflammatory Th17 cells and therapeutic implications. Mediators Inflamm 2015; 2015: 751793.
[http://dx.doi.org/10.1155/2015/751793] [PMID: 25918479]

[16]   Annunziato F, Cosmi L, Liotta F, Maggi E, Romagnani S. Type 17 T helper cells-origins, features and possible roles in rheumatic disease. Nat Rev Rheumatol 2009; 5(6): 325-31.
[http://dx.doi.org/10.1038/nrrheum.2009.80] [PMID: 19434074]

[17]   O'Shea JJ, Steward-Tharp SM, Laurence A, *et al.* Signal transduction and Th17 cell differentiation. Microbes Infect 2009; 11(5): 599-611.
[http://dx.doi.org/10.1016/j.micinf.2009.04.007] [PMID: 19379825]

[18]   Byng-Maddick R, Ehrenstein MR. The impact of biological therapy on regulatory T cells in rheumatoid arthritis. Rheumatology (Oxford) 2015; 54(5): 768-75.
[http://dx.doi.org/10.1093/rheumatology/keu487] [PMID: 25667434]

[19]   Chavele KM, Ehrenstein MR. Regulatory T-cells in systemic lupus erythematosus and rheumatoid arthritis. FEBS Lett 2011; 585(23): 3603-10.
[http://dx.doi.org/10.1016/j.febslet.2011.07.043] [PMID: 21827750]

[20]   Brink M, Hansson M, Mathsson L, *et al.* Multiplex analyses of antibodies against citrullinated peptides in individuals prior to development of rheumatoid arthritis. Arthritis Rheum 2013; 65(4): 899-910.
[http://dx.doi.org/10.1002/art.37835] [PMID: 23310951]

[21]   Tak PP, Gerlag DM, Aupperle KR, *et al.* Inhibitor of nuclear factor kappaB kinase beta is a key regulator of synovial inflammation. Arthritis Rheum 2001; 44(8): 1897-907.

[http://dx.doi.org/10.1002/1529-0131(200108)44:8<1897::AID-ART328>3.0.CO;2-4]   [PMID: 11508443]

[22]   Wang F, Sengupta TK, Zhong Z, Ivashkiv LB. Regulation of the balance of cytokine production and the signal transducer and activator of transcription (STAT) transcription factor activity by cytokines and inflammatory synovial fluids. J Exp Med 1995; 182(6): 1825-31.
[http://dx.doi.org/10.1084/jem.182.6.1825] [PMID: 7500028]

[23]   Lee DM, Kiener HP, Agarwal SK, *et al.* Cadherin-11 in synovial lining formation and pathology in arthritis. Science 2007; 315(5814): 1006-10.
[http://dx.doi.org/10.1126/science.1137306] [PMID: 17255475]

[24]   Lefèvre S, Knedla A, Tennie C, *et al.* Synovial fibroblasts spread rheumatoid arthritis to unaffected joints. Nat Med 2009; 15(12): 1414-20.
[http://dx.doi.org/10.1038/nm.2050] [PMID: 19898488]

[25]   Wisłowska M, Rok M, Jaszczyk B, Stepień K, Cicha M. Serum leptin in rheumatoid arthritis. Rheumatol Int 2007; 27(10): 947-54.
[http://dx.doi.org/10.1007/s00296-007-0335-4] [PMID: 17443329]

[26]   Redlich K, Hayer S, Ricci R, *et al.* Osteoclasts are essential for TNF-alpha-mediated joint destruction. J Clin Invest 2002; 110(10): 1419-27.
[http://dx.doi.org/10.1172/JCI0215582] [PMID: 12438440]

[27]   Harre U, Georgess D, Bang H, *et al.* Induction of osteoclastogenesis and bone loss by human autoantibodies against citrullinated vimentin. J Clin Invest 2012; 122(5): 1791-802.
[http://dx.doi.org/10.1172/JCI60975] [PMID: 22505457]

[28]   Brennan P, Barrett J, Fiddler M, Thomson W, Payton T, Silman A. Maternal-fetal HLA incompatibility and the course of inflammatory arthritis during pregnancy. J Rheumatol 2000; 27(12): 2843-8.
[PMID: 11128674]

[29]   Schellekens GA, de Jong BA, van den Hoogen FH, van de Putte LB, van Venrooij WJ. Citrulline is an essential constituent of antigenic determinants recognized by rheumatoid arthritis-specific autoantibodies. J Clin Invest 1998; 101(1): 273-81.
[http://dx.doi.org/10.1172/JCI1316] [PMID: 9421490]

[30]   van der Heijde D. Quantification of radiological damage in inflammatory arthritis: rheumatoid arthritis, psoriatic arthritis and ankylosing spondylitis. Best Pract Res Clin Rheumatol 2004; 18(6): 847-60.
[http://dx.doi.org/10.1016/j.berh.2004.05.007] [PMID: 15501186]

[31]   Arnett FC. Revised criteria for the classification of rheumatoid arthritis. Bull Rheum Dis 1989; 38(5): 1-6.
[PMID: 2679945]

[32]   Aletaha D, Neogi T, Silman AJ, *et al.* 2010 Rheumatoid arthritis classification criteria: an American College of Rheumatology/European League Against Rheumatism collaborative initiative. Arthritis Rheum 2010; 62(9): 2569-81.
[http://dx.doi.org/10.1002/art.27584] [PMID: 20872595]

[33]   Wisłowska M, Sypuła S, Kowalik I. Echocardiographic findings and 24-h electrocardiographic Holter monitoring in patients with nodular and non-nodular rheumatoid arthritis. Rheumatol Int 1999; 18(5-6): 163-9.
[http://dx.doi.org/10.1007/s002960050079] [PMID: 10399790]

[34]   Midtbø H, Semb AG, Matre K, Kvien TK, Gerdts E. Disease activity is associated with reduced left ventricular systolic myocardial function in patients with rheumatoid arthritis. Ann Rheum Dis 2017; 76(2): 371-6.
[http://dx.doi.org/10.1136/annrheumdis-2016-209223] [PMID: 27269296]

[35]   Ramey DR, Fries JF, Singh G. The Health Assessment Questionnaire 1995: status and review.Quality of life and pharmacoeconomics in clinical trials. 2nd ed. Philadelphia: Lippincott-Raven 1996; pp. 227-37.

[36]   Ware JE Jr, Sherbourne CD. The MOS 36-item short-form health survey (SF-36). I. Conceptual framework and item selection. Med Care 1992; 30(6): 473-83.
         [http://dx.doi.org/10.1097/00005650-199206000-00002] [PMID: 1593914]

[37]   Aletaha D, Smolen J. The Simplified Disease Activity Index (SDAI) and the Clinical Disease Activity Index (CDAI): a review of their usefulness and validity in rheumatoid arthritis. Clin Exp Rheumatol 2005; 23(5) (Suppl. 39): S100-8.
         [PMID: 16273793]

[38]   Van der Heijde DM. van t' Hof MA, van Riel PL, van de Putte LBA. Development of a disease activity score based on judgement in clinical practice by rheumatologists. J Rheumatol 1993; 20: 579-81.
         [PMID: 8478878]

[39]   Smolen JS, Breedveld FC, Eberl G, *et al.* Validity and reliability of the twenty-eight-joint count for the assessment of rheumatoid arthritis activity. Arthritis Rheum 1995; 38(1): 38-43.
         [http://dx.doi.org/10.1002/art.1780380106] [PMID: 7818569]

[40]   Fries JF, Spitz PW, Young DY. The dimensions of health outcomes: the health assessment questionnaire, disability and pain scales. J Rheumatol 1982; 9(5): 789-93.
         [PMID: 7175852]

[41]   Felson DT, Smolen JS, Wells G, *et al.* American College of Rheumatology/European League Against Rheumatism provisional definition of remission in rheumatoid arthritis for clinical trials. Arthritis Rheum 2011; 63(3): 573-86.
         [http://dx.doi.org/10.1002/art.30129] [PMID: 21294106]

[42]   van Gestel AM, Prevoo ML, van 't Hof MA, van Rijswijk MH, van de Putte LB, van Riel PL. Development and validation of the European League Against Rheumatism response criteria for rheumatoid arthritis. Comparison with the preliminary American College of Rheumatology and the World Health Organization/International League Against Rheumatism Criteria. Arthritis Rheum 1996; 39(1): 34-40.
         [http://dx.doi.org/10.1002/art.1780390105] [PMID: 8546736]

[43]   Smolen JS, Aletaha D, Bijlsma JW, *et al.* Treating rheumatoid arthritis to target: recommendations of an international task force. Ann Rheum Dis 2010; 69(4): 631-7.
         [http://dx.doi.org/10.1136/ard.2009.123919] [PMID: 20215140]

[44]   Grigor C, Capell H, Stirling A, *et al.* Effect of a treatment strategy of tight control for rheumatoid arthritis (the TICORA study): a single-blind randomised controlled trial. Lancet 2004; 364(9430): 263-9.
         [http://dx.doi.org/10.1016/S0140-6736(04)16676-2] [PMID: 15262104]

[45]   Visser K, Katchamart W, Loza E, *et al.* Multinational evidence-based recommendations for the use of methotrexate in rheumatic disorders with a focus on rheumatoid arthritis: integrating systematic literature research and expert opinion of a broad international panel of rheumatologists in the 3E Initiative. Ann Rheum Dis 2009; 68(7): 1086-93.
         [http://dx.doi.org/10.1136/ard.2008.094474] [PMID: 19033291]

[46]   Ostrov B, Robbins L. Improved tolerance and cost-effectiveness of subcutaneous vs. oral methotrexate in rheumatoid arthritis and juvenile rheumatoid arthritis. Arthritis Rheum 1998; 41 Suppl. 257.

[47]   Palmer G, Burger D, Mezin F, *et al.* The active metabolite of leflunomide, A77 1726, increases the production of IL-1 receptor antagonist in human synovial fibroblasts and articular chondrocytes. Arthritis Res Ther 2004; 6(3): R181-9.
         [http://dx.doi.org/10.1186/ar1157] [PMID: 15142263]

[48]   REMICADE ™ Rapidly reduces signs and symptoms of rheumatoid arthritis; ATTRACT study results positive on all endpoints. PR Newswire Association LLC; New York 1998; 1-3.

[49]   Klarenbeek NB, Güler-Yüksel M, van der Kooij SM, *et al.* The impact of four dynamic, goal-steered treatment strategies on the 5-year outcomes of rheumatoid arthritis patients in the BeSt study. Ann Rheum Dis 2011; 70(6): 1039-46.
[http://dx.doi.org/10.1136/ard.2010.141234] [PMID: 21415052]

[50]   Emery P, Breedveld FC, Hall S, *et al.* Comparison of methotrexate monotherapy with a combination of methotrexate and etanercept in active, early, moderate to severe rheumatoid arthritis (COMET): a randomised, double-blind, parallel treatment trial. Lancet 2008; 372(9636): 375-82.
[http://dx.doi.org/10.1016/S0140-6736(08)61000-4] [PMID: 18635256]

[51]   Klareskog L, van der Heijde D, de Jager JP, *et al.* Therapeutic effect of the combination of etanercept and methotrexate compared with each treatment alone in patients with rheumatoid arthritis: double-blind randomised controlled trial. Lancet 2004; 363(9410): 675-81.
[http://dx.doi.org/10.1016/S0140-6736(04)15640-7] [PMID: 15001324]

[52]   Weinblatt ME, Keystone EC, Furst DE, Kavanaugh AF, Chartash EK, Segurado OG. Long term efficacy and safety of adalimumab plus methotrexate in patients with rheumatoid arthritis: ARMADA 4 year extended study. Ann Rheum Dis 2006; 65(6): 753-9.
[http://dx.doi.org/10.1136/ard.2005.044404] [PMID: 16308341]

[53]   Hoff M, Kvien TK, Kälvesten J, Elden A, Haugeberg G. Adalimumab therapy reduces hand bone loss in early rheumatoid arthritis: explorative analyses from the PREMIER study. Ann Rheum Dis 2009; 68(7): 1171-6.
[http://dx.doi.org/10.1136/ard.2008.091264] [PMID: 18801760]

[54]   Emery P, Fleischmann RM, Strusberg I. Five-year safety and efficacy of golimumab in methotrexate-naïve patients with rheumatoid arthritis: final study results of the phase 3, randomized, placebo-controlled GO-BEFORE trial. Ann Rheum Dis 2013; 72: 432-7.
[http://dx.doi.org/10.1136/annrheumdis-2013-eular.1305]

[55]   Keystone E, Genovese MC, Klareskog L, *et al.* Golimumab in patients with active rheumatoid arthritis despite methotrexate therapy: 52-week results of the GO-FORWARD study. Ann Rheum Dis 2010; 69(6): 1129-35.
[http://dx.doi.org/10.1136/ard.2009.116319] [PMID: 20444749]

[56]   Smolen JS, Kay J, Doyle M, *et al.* Golimumab in patients with active rheumatoid arthritis after treatment with tumor necrosis factor α inhibitors: findings with up to five years of treatment in the multicenter, randomized, double-blind, placebo-controlled, phase 3 GO-AFTER study. Arthritis Res Ther 2015; 17: 14-21.
[http://dx.doi.org/10.1186/s13075-015-0516-6] [PMID: 25627338]

[57]   Haraoui B, Bykerk VP, Van Vollenhoven R. Long-term safety in rheumatoid arthritis before and after certolizumab pegol dose increase/decrease: analysis of data pooled from the RAPID1 and RAPID2 randomized trials (Report). Ann Rheum Dis 2014; 73: 929-36.
[http://dx.doi.org/10.1136/annrheumdis-2014-eular.1763]

[58]   Jones G, Sebba A, Gu J, *et al.* Comparison of tocilizumab monotherapy versus methotrexate monotherapy in patients with moderate to severe rheumatoid arthritis: the AMBITION study. Ann Rheum Dis 2010; 69(1): 88-96.
[http://dx.doi.org/10.1136/ard.2008.105197] [PMID: 19297346]

[59]   Van Vollenhoven R, Emery P, Fleischmann RM. Safety and tolerability of rituximab in patients with moderate to severe rheumatoid arthritis (RA): Results from the dose-ranging assessment international clinical evaluation of rituximab in RA (DANCER) study. Ann Rheum Dis 2005; 64: 432-7.

[60]   Kremer JM, Dougados M, Emery P, *et al.* Treatment of rheumatoid arthritis with the selective costimulation modulator abatacept: twelve-month results of a phase iib, double-blind, randomized, placebo-controlled trial. Arthritis Rheum 2005; 52(8): 2263-71.

[http://dx.doi.org/10.1002/art.21201] [PMID: 16052582]

[61]   O'Shea JJ, Schwartz DM, Villarino AV, Gadina M, McInnes IB, Laurence A. The JAK-STAT pathway: impact on human disease and therapeutic intervention. Annu Rev Med 2015; 66: 311-28.
       [http://dx.doi.org/10.1146/annurev-med-051113-024537] [PMID: 25587654]

CHAPTER 2

Spondyloarthropathies

Abstract: Spondyloarthropathies (SpA) are a group of chronic inflammatory arthropathies affecting the spine, sacroiliac joints, entheses and extra-articular sites. Clinical characteristics of spondyloarthritis are: peripheral arthritis, mainly in the lower limbs, asymmetrical, tendency for radiographic sacroilitis, no rheumatoid factor and presence of subcutaneous nodules. Significant familiar occurrence and association with HLA-B27 are characteristics for SpA. Diseases belonging to the group of spondyloarthritis are: ankylosing spondylitis, reactive arthritis (ReA), enteropathic arthritis (Crohn's disease, ulcerative colitis), psoriatic arthritis (PsA), undifferentiated spondyloarthritis and juvenile chronic arthritis (juvenile onset ankylosing spondylitis).

SpA occurs due to genetic predisposition especially in patients with positive test for major histocompatibility complex (MHC) class I molecule HLA-B27. Environmental factors are also involved in the pathogenesis. Extra-articular features include skin lesions in PsA, gut involvement in inflammatory bowel disease-related arthritis and the oculo-urethrosynovial triangle in ReA.

NSAIDs and anti TNFα drugs are effective in the treatment of axial manifestations of AS. Acute episodes of ReA are treated using NSAIDs and is used as the first line treatment. In more severe cases including NSAIDs resistance, systemic or prolonged disease, systemic GCS may be used. Management of peripheral arthritis in PsA: NSAIDs, GCS, DMARDS: MTX, or Sulfasalazine or Ciclosporin or Leflunomide, anti –TNFα, new options for treatment includes inhibitor IL-17 (ixekizumab or secukinumab), ustekinumab – a fully human IgG 1k monoclonal antibody that binds to the common p40 subunit shared by interleukins 12 and 23, and apremilast – a phosphodiesterase inhibitor.

Keywords: Ankylosing spondylitis (AS), Anterior uveitis, antiTNFα drugs, Apremilast, Asymmetrical, Crohn's disease, Entheses, HLA-B27, Ixekizumab, Lower limb, NSAIDs, Oculo-urethrosynovial triangle, Peripheral arthritis, Psoriatic arthritis (PsA), Reactive arthritis (ReA), Sacroiliac joints, Secukinumab, Spine, Spondyloarthropathies (SpA), Ulcerative colitis, Undifferentiated spondyloarthritis, Ustekinumab.

INTRODUCTION

Spondyloarthropathies (SpA) are a group of chronic inflammatory arthropathies targeting the spine, entheses and extra-articular sites. Clinical features of spondy-

Małgorzata Wisłowska

loarthritis are: peripheral arthritis, mainly in the lower limb, asymmetrical, tendency for radiographic sacroilitis, no rheumatoid factor and presence of subcutaneous nodules. Significant familiar occurrence and association with HLA-B27 are characteristic for SpA. Diseases belonging to the group of spondyloarthritis are: ankylosing spondylitis, reactive arthritis (ReA), enteropathic arthritis (Crohn's disease, ulcerative colitis), psoriatic arthritis (PsA), undifferentiated spondyloarthritis and juvenile chronic arthritis (juvenile onset ankylosing spondylitis).

SpA occurs due to genetic predisposition especially in patients with a positive test for the major histocompatibility complex (MHC) class I molecule HLA-B27. Environmental factors are also involved in the pathogenesis.

Clinical features of SpA include inflammation of the spine and sacroiliac joints, peripheral arthritis and enthesitis (inflammation at the entheses, the sites of attachment of tendons, ligaments, fasciae or joint capsules to bone). Extra-articular features include skin lesions in PsA, gut involvement in enteropathic arthritis and the oculo-urethrosynovial triangle in ReA.

The first clinical symptom is back pain, occurring in 75% of patients with axial SpA. The dull pain begins in the lumbar region or at the lumbosacral junction, becoming constant after a few months and is accompanied with morning stiffness lasting for more than 30 minutes. It improves after physical activity and non-steroidal anti-inflammatory drugs (NSAIDs). The pain can also occur during the night. X-ray revealing sacroilitis or spondylitis with ankylosis.

Three criteria of inflammatory back pain with similar sensitivities and specificities have been proposed.

The first one is CALIN inflammatory back pain criteria [1].

At least four of the following criteria:

1. Insidious onset
2. Onset before the age of 40 years
3. At least 3 months' duration
4. Morning stiffness about 30 minutes
5. Improvement with exercise

If four of these five criteria are fulfilled, sensitivity is 95% and specificity is 85% [1].

The second one is BERLIN inflammatory back pain criteria [2].

At least two of the following criteria:

1. Morning stiffness equal or more than 30 minutes
2. Improvement with exercise but not with rest
3. Disrupted sleep due to back pain
4. Alternating buttock pain

If two of these four criteria are fulfilled, sensitivity is 70% and specificity is 81%. If three out of four criteria are fulfilled, sensitivity is 83% and specificity is 98% [2].

The third one is EXPERT criteria for inflammatory back pain [3].

1. Improvement with exercise
2. Pain at night
3. Insidious onset
4. Age at onset before 40 years
5. No improvement with rest

The criteria are fulfilled if at least four of these five criteria are met [3].

ANKYLOSING SPONDYLITIS (AS)

Ankylosing spondylitis is currently known as spondyloarthritis and is the main type of axial SpA. It is characterised by pain in the spine, limitation in spinal mobility and radiological changes in the sacroiliac joints and the spine. Enthesitis is observed in 40-60% of cases and acute anterior uveitis in 30-50% of cases. The disease is characterised by chronic axial inflammation with restricted mobility of the spine and decreased function. Diagnosis is often delayed up to 5 to 10 years due to the need for X-ray evidence of abnormalities of the sacroiliac joints. During this period many patients undergo unnecessary investigations and receive inappropriate treatment.

The term "axial spondyloarthritis" (or axial spondyloarthropathy) is more inclusive and includes ankylosing spondylitis. The diagnosis of axial spondyloarthritis can be based just on clinical symptoms even before X-ray. MRI shows sacroiliac joint inflammation years before any evidence on X-rays pictures.

The prevalence of ankylosing spondylitis (AS) is between 0.1% and 1%, with a male predominance of 2-3: 1. The geographical distribution represents the frequency of HLA-B27 in the population.

Inflammation starts in the sacroiliac joints causing "alternating buttock pain" and later involves the spine, causing back pain and stiffness. The disease begins in late adolescence and early adulthood. Pain worsens with physical inactivity and is eased with exercise, a hot shower, or the use of NSAIDs.

Some patients may present with extra articular features, such as acute iritis, psoriasis or inflammatory bowel disease.

Involvement of the thoracic spine, the costovertebral and costotransverse joints, paravertebral ligaments and anterior chest wall causes chest pain which worsens with coughing or sneezing.

An early diagnosis is important as it is now possible to treat patients with more effective therapies such as TNF antagonists. These drugs are more effective in early stages of the disease.

A positive genetic test for HLA B27 may confirm the diagnosis of axial spondyloarthritis if the clinical picture suggests this diagnosis but there are no findings on imaging studies.

Pathogenesis

The etiology of SpA is unknown but probably includes genetic and environmental factors. The importance of genetic factors in developing AS has been shown due to frequent familial occurrence in cases.

The first genetic factor was the tissue antigen HLA-B27. Other genes important in disease susceptibility are different B27 subtypes and non-B27 MHC and non-MHC genes.

HLA-B27 heavy chains form homodimers without beta2-microglobulin light chain, which can be targeted by proinflammatory responses.

Non-B27 MHC Genes. The MHC consists of around 220 genes, which may have immunoregulatory functions and may be involved in pathogenesis of AS.

Non-MHC Genes Associated with AS. The study was carried out by the Wellcome Trust Case Consortium and the Australo-Anglo-American Spondyloarthritis Consortium (TASC, 2010) [4]. In the study, 14 500 non-synonymous SNPs (*i.e.* SNPs which change the amino acid sequence) identified disease association with interleukin 23 receptor (IL-23R) and endoplasmic reticulum amino-peptidase 1 (ERAP1). IL-23R has also been linked with IBD and PsA [4].

Infections. Several gastrointestinal or genitourinary pathogens which are confirmed by DNA polymerase chain reactions in synovial cell and fluid are associated with ReA.

AS begins with entheses, the site of attachment of ligaments, tendons and capsules to bone. Later, as can cause bone erosion and syndesmophytes which joint the vertebral bodies into a single unit, so-called "bamboo spine".

Besides HLA- B27, TNF alpha, IL-1 beta, IL-6 and IL-23/17 are involved in the pathogenesis of AS. IL-23 activates JAK2 and STAT3 signaling pathway. Overexpression of IL-23 causes axial and peripheral enthesitis, sacroilitis with syndesmophyte, aortic root and valve inflammation.

Spondylitis causes ankylosis of the axial skeleton, which results from ossification of the ligaments, costovertebral and sternocostal joints. The first sign of an abnormal posture is the loss of lumbar lordosis, followed by thoracic hyperkyphosis. Spinal movement is restricted.

Anterior chest wall pain occurs in about 15% of patients and is due to sternoclavicular, manubriosternal and sternocostal arthritis. It can cause reduced chest expansion.

Arthritis of the hips and shoulders affects 1/3 of patients. Hip involvement is commonly bilateral and leads to severe disability.

Peripheral arthritis is typically asymmetrical, oligoarticular and involves the lower limbs. Upper limb involvement is connected with PsA. A bilateral symmetrical polyarticular involvement is observed but without positive rheumatoid factor. The distal interphalangeal joints are also affected in PsA. This differs PsA with RA.

Dactylitis (sausage finger) is a characteristic for SpA. It is typical for ReA, PsA or undifferentiated SpA. The swelling involves the whole finger (sausage finger).

Modified New York Criteria for Ankylosing Spondylitis (1984) [5]

Clinical Criteria

a. Low back pain for at least 3 months duration improved by exercise and not relieved by rest
b. Limitation of lumbar spine motion in sagital and frontal planes
c. Chest expansion decreased relative to normal values for age and sex.

Radiological Criterion

Sacroilitis grade >2 bilaterally or grade 3-4 unilaterally.

Definite ankylosing spondylitis if the radiological criterion is associated with at least 1 clinical criterion.

The European Spondylarthropathy Study Group (ESSG) Classification Criteria for Spondyloarthropathy (SpA) [6]

Inflammatory back pain or synovitis plus one of the following:

• Enthesitis (heel)
• Positive family history
• Psoriasis
• Crohn's disease, ulcerative colitis
• Urethritis (cervicitis or acute diarrhea within one month before arthritis)
• Buttock pain (alternating between right and left gluteal areas)
• Sacroilitis.
• The sensitivity of these criteria is 62.5%, and specificity 81.1%.

Amor Classification Criteria for Spondyloarthritis [7]

a. Clinical Symptoms/History Score
   1. Pain at night (spine) or morning stiffness 1.
   2. Asymmetrical oligoarthritis 2.
   3. Gluteal (buttock) pain (any) or 1.
   4. Alternating gluteal pain 2.
   5. Sausage like digit or toe (dactylitis) 2.
   6. Enthesitis (heel) 2.
   7. Uveitis 2.
   8. Urethritis/Cervicitis within 1 month before onset of arthritis 1.
   9. Diarrhea within 1 month before onset of arthritis 1.
   10. Psoriasis, balanitis or inflammatory bowel disease 2.
b. X-rays
   Sacroilitis (grade 2 bilateraly or grade 3 unilateraly) 3.
c. Genetical background
   HLA-B27 positive or positive family history for AS, ReA, uveitis, psoriasis or inflammatory bowel disease 2.
d. Good response to non-steroidal anti-inflammatory drugs (NSAIDs)
   NSAIDs show a good response within 48 hours, or relapse within 48 hours after NSAIDs are stopped 2.
   The sensitivity of these criteria is 39.8% and specificity is 97.8%.

ASAS Classification criteria for axial spondyloarthritis (SpA) 2009 [8]

In patients with >3 months of back pain and age <45 ys.

Sacroilitis on imaging plus ≥1 SpA feature

or HLA-B27 ≥2 other SpA features.

Sacroilitis on imaging:

• Active (acute) inflammation on MRI highly suggestive of sacroilitis associated
  with SpA
• Definite radiographic sacroilitis according to mod. NY criteria.

SpA features:

inflammatory back pain, arthritis, enthesitis (heel), uveitis, dactylitis, psoriasis,
Crohn's/colitis, good response to (non-steroidal anti-inflammatory drugs)
NSAIDs, family history for SpA, HLA-B27 and elevated CRP.

The sensitivity of these criteria is 82.9% and specificity is 84.4%.

ASAS Classification criteria for peripheral spondyloarthritis (SpA) 2011 [9]

Arthritis or enthesitis or dactylitis plus

≥1 SpA feature or ≥ other SpA features

Uveitis	Arthritis
Psoriasis	Enthesitis
Crohn's/colitis	Dactylitis
Preceding infection	Inflammatory back pain
HLA-B27	Family history for SpA.

Sacroilitis in imaging

The sensitivity of these criteria is 79.5% and specificity is 83.3%.

Association with psoriasis, chronic inflammatory bowel disease and reactive
arthritis may occur in some patients with AS. Patients respond well to anti-
inflammatory doses of NSAIDs. Extra-articular features of ankylosing spondylitis
are: iritis, impaired lung function, upper lobe fibrosis, aortic incompetence,
cardiac conduction defects, spinal cord, root compression and amyloidosis.

Measurement of disease outcome in AS
Disease Activity

Bath Ankylosing Spondylitis Disease Activity Index (BASDAI) [10]

Fatigue/tired	0 – 10
Neck/back/hip pain	0 – 10
Other joint pain	0 – 10
Touch discomfort	0 – 10
Morning stiffness	0 – 10
Morning stiffness	HR - MIN

BASDAI is used as an instrument to measure disease activity in AS. These individual values are added and the result is divided by six. The result more than four is a high activity of disease patient and Physician Global Assessment.

Ankylosing Spondylitis Disease Activity Score (ASDAS) [11]

Back pain	0 – 10
Duration morning stiffness	0 – 10
Patient global	0 – 10
Peripheral pain/swelling	0 – 10
CRP (mg/l)	
ESR (mm/hr)	
ASDAS – CRP	
ASDAS - ESR	

The Ankylosing Spondylitis Disease Activity Score (ASDAS) is a new index used to assess disease activity. It combines five disease activity variables with partial overlap, resulting in one score which is more valid, with improved sensitivity to change compared to single-item variables. There are the two ASDAS formulas:

1. ASDAS-CRP - 0.12 x Back Pain + 0.06x Duration of Morning Stiffness + 0.11 x Patient Global + 0.07 x Peripheral Pain/Swelling + 0.58 x Ln (CRP + 1)
2. ASDAS-ESR – 0.08 x Back Pain + 0.07 x Duration of Morning Stiffness + 0.11 x Patient Global + 0.09 x Peripheral Pain/Swelling + 0.29 x V(ESR)

V(ESR) – square root of the erythrocyte sedimentation rate (mm/h)

Ln (CRP+ 1) – natural logarithm of the C-reactive protein (mg/L) +1

Back pain, patient global, duration of morning stiffness and peripheral pain/swelling are all assessed on a visual scale (from 0 to 10 cm) or on a numerical rating scale (from 0 to 10).

Back pain, BASDAI question 2: "How would you describe the overall level of AS neck, back or hip pain you have had?".

Duration of morning stiffness, BASDAI question 6: " How long does your morning stiffness last from the time you wake up?".

Patient global: "How active was your spondylitis on average during the last week?".

Peripheral pain/swelling, BASDAI question 3: "How would you describe the overall level of pain/swelling in joints other than neck, back or hips you have had?".

The Assessment of SpondyloArthritis International Society (ASAS) membership has selected the ASDAS containing C-reactive protein (CRP, mg/l) as acute phase reactant as the preferred version, and the one with erythrocyte sedimentation rate (ESR, mm/hr) as the alternative version. Apart from the value of CRP or ESR, the four additional self-reported items included in this index are back pain (0- 10 cm, visual analogue scale [VAS] or 0-10, numerical rating scale [NRS], duration of morning stiffness (VAS/NRS), peripheral pain/swelling (VAS/NRS) and patient global assessment of disease activity (VAS/NRS).

ASDAS is used as an instrument to measure disease activity in AS. The 3 cut-offs selected to separate these states were: < 1.3 between "inactive disease" and "moderate disease activity", < 2.1 between "moderate disease activity" and "high disease activity", and > 3.5 between "high disease activity" and "very high disease activity".

Function

Bath Ankylosing Spondylitis Functional Index (BASFI) [12]

Put on socks	0 – 10
Bind up wrist	0 – 10
Reach up shelf	0 – 10
Rise from chair	0 – 10
Rise from lying	0 – 10
Stand 10 min.	0 – 10
Climb 12 steps	0 – 10
Look over shoulder	0 – 10
Physical activity	0 – 10
Work all day	0 – 10

Health Assessment Questionnaire Spondylitis (HAQ-S) [13]

Metrometry

Schober test (lumbar flexion)

Chest expansion

Occiput-to-wall distance

Lateral bending

Bath Ankylosing Spondylitis Metrometry Index

Quality of life

Medical Outcome Study Short Form-36 (MOS-SF-36)

Ankylosing Spondylitis Quality of Life Index.

The Columna Vertebrae

The Cervical Spine – Flexion, extension, right lateral flexion, left lateral flexion, left rotation, right rotation. Occiput-wall distance – appropriate measurement of the distance from the wall to the occiput.

The Thoracic Spine – In order to check the mobility of the thoracic spine the Otto test is performed. 30 cm is measured down from C7 and the end points are marked. Next, the patient is asked to bend forward and try to touch the floor, the distance between the marked points is measured again. Usually the registered difference is between 2-3 cm.

The Lumbar Spine – Patients are asked to bend forward and touch the floor. The distance between the top of the third finger and the floor is measured – this is known as the Thomayer test. The normal value is 0. This test assesses global flexibility of the thoracic and lumbar spine.

Chest expansion can be measured by asking the patients to breath in and out and the difference between these two parameters is recorded. The normal value is between 5 to 12 cm.

The mobility of the lumbar spine is measured by performing the Schober test. From L5, 10 cm is measured up. Next, the patient is asked to bend forward and the distance is checked again; the difference between the first and the second measurement is around 5 cm.

Patrick's test – The patient's hip and ankle flexibility are tested to certain regions of pain. The usual locations of pain during this test are expressed as changes in the sacroiliac joints.

Imaging

Standard radiographs

Computer tomography

Bath Ankylosing Spondylitis Radiographic Index

Modified Stokes Ankylosing Spondylitis Scoring System

Magnetic resonance imaging.

Radiographic changes characteristic of spondyloarthropathies include normal bone mineralization, erosion, periostitis and bone proliferation at entheses.

X-rays of spine, sacroiliac joints and peripheral joints can show structural changes, but they are not visible in the early, "non-radiographic" stage.

Radiographic sacroilitis is the characteristic of AS and takes several years to become visible on plain radiographs. The earliest visible changes are blurring of the cortical margins of the subchondral bone, erosions and sclerosis. Joint changes usually become symmetrical. Radiographic sacroilitis can be graded according to the New York grading system as follows:

Grade I – suspicious

Grade II – evidence of erosion and sclerosis

Grade III – erosions, sclerosis and early ankylosis

Grade IV – total ankylosis.

Ankylosing spondylitis – bilateral symmetrical involvement of sacroiliac joints with early ankylosis, symmetrical syndesmophytes and peripheral involvement of shoulders and hips.

X-ray changes of the spine show squaring of the vertebrae. Vertebral enthesitis may cause sclerosis of the upper and lower vertebral bodies. Annulus fibrous ossification leads to syndesmophyte formation which results in a "bamboo spine".

Reactive arthritis – bilateral asymmetrical sacroiliac involvement, bulky asymmetrical paravertebral ossification and typical involvement of lower extremity joints.

Psoriatic arthritis – spinal and sacroiliac changes similar to reactive arthritis and common involvement of wrists, hands, feet and shoulders.

MRI can detect inflammatory lesions long before changes can be observed on plain radiographs.

To recognise "sacroilitis by MRI" the following features must be met according to ASA/OMERACT [14]:

1. Active inflammatory lesions of the sacroiliac joints, BMO (on STIR) or osteitis (on T1 after Gd) must be clearly located in typical anatomical areas (subchondral or periarticular bone marrow)
2. When a single BMO lesion is observed, this should be present on at least two consecutive slices
3. When more BMO lesions are observed on one slice, documentation of inflammation by using a single slice is enough
4. The presence of synovitis, enthesitis or capsulitis without concomitant BMO/osteitis is not sufficient enough for diagnosis.

A definition of a "positive" MRI of the spine has also been proposed by ASAS. Acording to this definition, evidence of spondylitis in three or more vertebral sites is highly suggestive of inflammatory lesions related to axSpA, while evidence of fatty deposition in several sites (at least 5) is highly suggestive of postinflammatory lesion-related axSpA. These lesions should be located at the edges of the vertebrae, regardless of whether these edges are in the anterior or the posterior part of the vertebral body.

The Pathophysiological Role of B27 in AS

Altered pathogen interactions are associated with aberrant antigenic processing of self-proteins, which could include B27 itself following misfolding of the heavy chain and retrograde transport from the endoplasmic reticulum. B27 restricted presentation of an arthritogenic self-peptides may trigger the activation of cytotoxic T cells through cross-reactivity with bacterial peptides.

Management of Ankylosing Spondylitis

Management of ankylosing spondylitis includes patient education and physical therapy. Physical therapy maintains posture and movement to near normal. Exercises must be continued throughout life. Regular exercises are effective in reducing pain and preserving function. Supervised exercises are more effective than home exercises.

In cases with hip involvement, severe spinal deformity or vertebral fractures, surgery is required.

NSAIDs, anti TNFα anti IL-17 drugs are drugs of choice for treatment of axial manifestations of AS. NSAIDs relieve pain and stiffness and are effective in preventing radiological progression.

Genome-wide association studies in AS have shown an association of the gene prostaglandin receptor 4 (*PTGER4*) with AS. Bone resorption can be affected by the *PTGER* gene and this effect may be modified by NSAIDs. *PTGER4* can induce bone formation in fatty areas of the marrow using adipose tissue and therefore, is a potential key factor involved in syndesmophyte formation. Prostaglandins can also stimulate osteoblast formation. Differences in local concentrations of prostaglandins could explain the paradoxical new bone formation and osteoporosis in AS. The inhibition of new bone formation by NSAIDs can be explained by the inhibition of prostaglandin (especially prostaglandin E2) synthesis mediated by COX-2.

Monoarticular or oligoarticular arthritis is treated by intra-articular GCS injections. Oral GCS improves peripheral synovitis, but are not effective in axial diseases.

Sulfasalazine and MTX are used in cases of peripheral joint involvement. Anti-TNFα therapy is very effective in improving disease progression. Anti-IL-17 agents like brodalumab, ixekizumab and secukinumab – all monoclonal antibodies targeting the IL-17 pathway are introduced to treatment after failure when using TNF inhibitors.

2016 update of the ASAS-EULAR Management Recommendations for Axial Spondyloarthritis [15]

Overarching principles:

1. axSpA is a potentially severe disease with diverse manifestations, usually requiring multidisciplinary management coordinated by the rheumatologist.

2. The primary goal of treating the patient with axSpA is to maximise health-related quality of life through control of symptoms and inflammation, prevention of progressive structural damage, preservation/ normalisation of function and social participation.

3. The optimal management of patients with axSpA requires a combination of

non-pharmacological and pharmacological treatment modalities.

4. Treatment of axSpA should aim at the best care and must be based on a shared decision between the patient and the rheumatologist.

5. axSpA involves high individual, medical and social costs, all of which should be considered in its management by the treating rheumatologist.

Recommendations:

1. The treatment of patients with axSpA should be individualised according to the current signs and symptoms of the disease (axial, peripheral, extra-articular manifestations) and the patient characteristics including comorbidities and psychological factors.

2. Disease monitoring of patients with axSpA should include patient-reported outcomes, clinical findings, laboratory tests and imaging, all with the appropriate instruments and relevant to the clinical presentation. The frequency of monitoring should be decided on an individual basis depending on symptoms, severity and treatment.

3. Treatment should be guided according to a predefined treatment target.

4. Patients should be educated about axSpA and encouraged to exercise on a regular basis and stop smoking; physical therapy should be considered.

5. Patients suffering from pain and stiffness should use an NSAID as first-line drug treatment up to maximum dose, taking risk and benefits into account. For patients who respond well to NSAIDs continous use is preferred, if symptomatic otherwise.

6. Analgesics, such as paracetamol and opioid-(like) drugs, might be considered for residual pain after previously recommended treatments have failed, are contraindicated and/or poorly tolerated.

7. Glucocorticoid injections directed to the local site of musculoskeletal inflammation may be considered. Patients with axial disease should not receive long-term treatment with systemic glucocorticoids.

8. Patients with purely axial disease should normally not be treated with csDMARDs; sulfasalazine may be considered in patients with peripheral arthritis.

9. bDMARDs should be considered in patients with persistently high disease activity despite conventional treatments; current practice is to start with TNFi

therapy.

10. If TNFi fails, switching to another TNFi or IL-17i therapy should be considered.

11. If a patient is in sustained remission, tapering of a bDMARD can be considered.

12. Total hip arthroplasty should be considered in patients with refractory pain or disability and radiographic evidence of structural damage, independent of age; spinal corrective osteotomy in specialised centres may be considered in patients with severe disabling deformity.

13. If a significant change in the course of the disease occurs, cases other than inflammation, such as a spinal fracture, should be considered and appropriate evaluation, including imaging, should be performed.

REACTIVE ARTHRITIS

Reactive arthritis (ReA) is an acute aseptic inflammatory arthritis, with or without extraarticular lesions, that develop after infection at a distant site. ReA occurs 1-month after an infection. Usually, it is after a genitourinary tract infection with Chlamydia trachomatis or enteritis infection with Gram-negative enterobacteria such as Shigella, Salmonella, Yersinia or Campylobacter species.

In developed countries, the cause of ReA is Chlamydia trachomatis, but in developing countries, the cause is after infections with enterobacteria. However, in about 25% of cases, the bacteria is unknown. Bacteria that trigger reactive arthritis are: Chlamydia trachomatis, Shigella flexneri, Salmonella species, Yersinia enterocolitica, Yersinia pseudotuberculosis, Campylobacter fetus jejuni, Clostridium difficile and Chlamydia pneumonia.

The interaction of host HLA-B27 and bacteria in the pathogenesis of spondyloarthropathies is very important. The process was initiated by specific bacterial infections in the gastrointestinal or genital tract, possibly in the upper respiratory tract and other locations. Susceptibility to the disease is strongly linked to possession of the HLA-B27 antigen.The spondyloarthropathies may be triggered by CD8+ T cells responding to peptides derived from bacteria which are bound to HLA-B27.

The classic ReA is the triad of arthritis, conjunctivitis and urethritis. ReA is typically an acute, asymmetrical oligoarthritis and is associated with extra-articular features, such as ocular inflammation (conjunctivitis or acute iritis), enthesitis, mucocutaneous lesions, urethritis and uncommonly with carditis.

Conjunctivitis occurs in one-third of patients, usually at the same time as arthritis, and acute anterior uveitis may occur at some time in about 5% of patients. The average duration of arthritis is 4-5 months. About 15-30% of patients develop chronic or recurrent peripheral arthritis, sacroilitis or spondylitis. Most patients with chronic ReA have a family member with SpA or are HLA-B27 positive.

Key features: Lower limb arthritis, enthesopathy, tendinitis, dactylitis, psoriasiform skin and mucous membrane lesions, eye lesions, notably anterior uveitis and conjunctivitis. Visceral involvement, such as nephritis or carditis, is rare and severity may be mild arthralgia to disabling disease. Recovery is usually spontaneous and the prognosis is good, however recurrence is common. A minority of patients may go on to develope ankylosing spondylitis.

REITER'S SYNDROME – An episode of peripheral arthritis of more than 1 month duration occurring in association with conjunctivitis, urethritis and/or cervicitis. Circinate balanitis and keratoderma blenorrhagica are also observed.

MANAGEMENT

Most patients are young, healthy adults whose disease are likely to resolve or improve spontaneously.

Acute episodes are treated using NSAIDs and usually, they are the first line treatment.

In more severe cases including NSAIDs resistance, systemic or prolonged disease, systemic GCS may be used. GCS may be administered as a single intra-muscular dose of depot methylprednisolone (80-120 mg), especially if a second line drug is being introduced, or as a course of oral prednisolone (15-30 mg once daily), the dose being tapered according to response. GCS therapy should be used for the shortest possible period of time and accompanied by appropriate bone protective treatment. Joint injection with GCS may improve the symptoms.

The second line drug is Sulfasalazine which is effective for peripheral arthritis. Azathioprine and other DMARDs have been used in patients with severe reactive arthritis.

The potential value of medium to long term (3-12 months) antimicrobial therapy in reactive arthritis with doxycycline, ciprofloxacin and azithromycin were observed. However, neither treatment was effective for arthritis. In cases of Chlamydia trachomatis infection in the urogenital tract, treatment with an antibiotic for 10-14 days is administered to prevent arthritis.

PSORIATIC ARTHRITIS

Psoriatic arthritis (PsA) is an inflammatory arthritis associated with psoriasis, without the presence of rheumatoid factor. Prevalence is 0.04-0.1%, however prevalence of psoriasis is 1-3% among Caucasian and only 0-0.3% among Afro-Caribben and Native American populations. About 10-20% of patients with psoriasis have PsA. Nail changes have the strongest association with arthropathy, particularly affecting the distal interphalangeal joints. The arthritis begins between 30 and 50 years of age, but may also occur in childhood.

The genetic susceptibility for PsA is polygenic. PsA is associated with genes that are associated with psoriasis (*e.g.* HLA-Cw6) and with arthritis (*e.g.* HLA-B27). A newly recognized class-I-related gene A (*MICA*) is more strongly associated with PsA itself and correlates with the susceptibility for developing PsA. Environmental factors which may trigger developing PsA are infection, trauma and stress.

Psoriatic arthritis is a systemic disease that can lead to chronic pain and loss of function. The main clinical symptoms are psoriasis, peripheral arthritis, axial disease, enthesitis and dactylitis or "sausage finger". The involvement of joints may be asymmetrical with dactylitis. A few patients present with arthritis of the distal interphalangeal joints, called "arthritis mutilans".

In X-rays, there are juxtra-articular new bone formation, absence of periarticular osteopenia and relative preservation of the joint space.

CASPAR Classification Criteria for Psoriatic Arthritis [16]

Active current psoriasis – score 2

A history of psoriasis (in the absence of current psoriasis) – score 1

A family history of psoriasis in a first- or second-degree relative (in the absence of current psoriasis and history of psoriasis) – score 1

Dactylitis – score 1

Juxta-articular new-bone formation – score 1

Rheumatoid factor negativity – score 1

Nail dystrophy – score 1

The patient is considered to have PsA if the sum of the points is ≥3 [16].

PSORIASIS: Psoriasis Area Severity Index (PASI) [17] and Short form (SF) 36
NAIL DISEASE: Nail Assessment in Psoriasis (NAPSI) [18], Psoriatic Nail
Severity Index (NPSS) [18].

A few scales were developed in order to evaluate the degree of psoriatic
progression in the nails, including: NAPSI, mNAPSI and PNSS. In the Psoriasis
Nail Severity Score (PNSS) [18] scale, one point is given for the presence of each
change from the following list: pitting, subungual hyperkeratosis, onycholysis and
advanced deformation of both nail ends. The maximum score is 4 for a nail.

The Nail Psoriasis Severity Index (NAPSI) scale grades the psoriatic changes of
the nails differently – the nail is divided with imaginary horizontal and
longitudinal lines into quadrants. Each nail is given a score for bed nail lesions
(0-4 points) and nail matrices (0-4 points) depending on the presence of any of the
features in that quadrant. Nail matrix psoriasis is characterized by nail plate
changes of pitting, leukonychia, red spots in the lunula and nail plate crumbling.
Nail bed psoriasis shows onycholysis, oil-drop dyschromia, splinter hemorrhages
and subungual hyperkeratosis. Thus, for each nail, the NAPSI score can amount to
8 points. As an alternative, a target nail can be selected and graded by means of
evaluation for the presence of all 8 criteria in each quadrant of the nail with total
sum of 32 points.

Modified Nail Psoriasis Severity Index (mNAPSI) scale also takes into account all
8 psoriatic changes of the nail without dividing it into parts, and the oil-drop
syndrome and the onycholysis are combined together in one criterion.
Additionally, in nail evaluation by using mNAPSI scale lesions: oil-drop
dyschromia/onycholysis and dystrophy are graded from 1 to 3 in terms of
severity. The presence of others are scored for 1 point. The maximum sum is 13
points for each nail. mNAPSI scale is considered to be an objective, numeric,
reproducible grading system of nail psoriasis with a relatively simple algorithm of
evaluation [18].

PERIPHERAL JOINTS: Modified ACR 20/50/70 criteria, Psoriatic Arthritis
Response Criteria (PsARC) and Disease Activity Score (DAS) 28 [19].

AXIAL SKELETON: Bath Ankylosing Spondylitis Disease Activity (BASDAI)
score [10] and Ankylosing Spondylitis Activity Score (ASAS) [11].

ENTHESITIS: Mander Index and Mastricht Ankylosing Spondylitis Score
(MASES) [20].

Management of Peripheral Arthritis

- Non-steroidal anti-inflammatory drugs

- GCS (dermatologist avoids the use of chronic oral GCS in psoriasis because discontinuation is often followed by a flare of the underlying skin disease or the development of pustular psoriasis).

- DMARDS: MTX – 15-20 mg/week (patients with PsA on MTX are more likely to develop histological progression of liver fibrosis than RA patients) or Sulfasalazine 3.0 g/day or Ciclosporin 3-5 mg/kg/day or Leflunomide 20 mg/day.

- Anti –TNFα treatment is effective in PsA and leads to a reduction in synovitis and psoriatic lesions. The magnitude and the time course of the effect on both symptoms demonstrate the pathogenic role of this cytokine in PsA. In PsA besides TNFα inhibitors, new options for treatment include inhibitor IL-17 (ixekizumab secukinumab), ustekinumab – a fully human IgG 1k monoclonal antibody that binds to the common p40 subunit shared by interleukins 12 and 23 and apremilast – a phosphodiesterase inhibitor.

2016 EULAR Recommendation for the Management of psoriatic Arthritis [21]

Overarching Principles

A. PsA is a heterogeneous and potentially severe disease, which may require multidisciplinary treatment.

B. Treatment of patients with PsA should aim at the best care and must be based on a shared decision between the patient and the rheumatologist, considering efficacy, safety and costs.

C. Rheumatologists are the specialists who should primarily care for the musculoskeletal manifestations of patients with PsA; in the presence of clinically significant skin involvement a rheumatologist and a dermatologist should collaborate in diagnosis and management.

D. The primary goal of treating patients with PsA is to maximize health-related quality of life; through control of symptoms, prevention of structural damage, normalization of function and social participation; decreasing inflammation is an important component to achieve these goals.

E. When managing patients with PsA, extra-articular manifestations, metabolic syndrome, cardiovascular disease and other comorbidities should be taken into account.

RECOMMENDATIONS

1. Treatment should be aimed at reaching remission or, alternatively, minimal/ low disease activity, by regular monitoring and appropriate adjustment of therapy.

2. In patients with PsA, NSAIDs may be used to relieve musculoskeletal signs and symptoms.

3. In patients with peripheral arthritis, particularly in those with many swollen joints, structural damage in the presence of inflammation, high ESR/ CRP and/ or clinically relevant extra-articular manifestations, csDMARDs should be considered at an early stage, with methotrexate preferred in those with relevant skin involvement.

4. Local injections of glucocorticoids should be considered as adjunctive therapy in PsA, systemic glucocorticoids may be used with caution at the lowest effective dose.

5. In patients with peripheral arthritis and an inadequate response to at least one csDMARD, therapy with a bDMARD, usually a TNF inhibitor, should be initiated.

6. In patients with peripheral arthritis and an inadequate response to at least one csDMARD, in whom TNF inhibitors are not appropriate, bDMARD targeting IL12/23 or IL17 pathways may be considered.

7. In patients with peripheral arthritis and an inadequate response to at least one csDMARD, where bDMARD are not appropriate, a targeted synthetic DMARD such as a PDE4-inhibitor may be considered.

8. In patients with active enthesitis and/or dactilitis and a poor response to NSAIDs or local glucocorticoid injections, therapy with a bDMARDs should be considered, which according to current practice is a TNF inhibitor.

9. In patients with predominantly axial disease that is active and has a poor response to NSAIDs, therapy with a bDMARDs should be considered, which according to current practice is a TNF inhibitor.

10. In patients who fail to respond adequately to a bDMARD, switching to another bDMARD should be considered, including switching between TNF inhibitors.

ENTEROPATHIC ARTHRITIS

Enteropathic arthritis is an inflammatory arthritis in patients with ulcerative colitis (UC) or Crohn's disease (CD). The prevalence of arthritis in enteropathic arthritis ranges from 17% to 20%, with a higher prevalence in CD.

The most common symptoms of enteropathic arthritis are arthritis of the knee and ankle joints, which are transient, migratory and non-deforming. The inflammatory episodes are self-limiting. Axial involvement and enthesitis may be present. Sometimes arthritis is chronic and destructive.

The treatment of peripheral arthritis in patients with enteropathic arthritis is the same as for other SpA, but NSAIDs should be administered with care as they may exacerbate intestinal symptoms.

Some patients with SpA have subclinical microscopic inflammatory gut lesions such as in Crohn disease. Chronic use of NSAIDs can lead to ulcerations of the gastrointestinal system.

Intra-articuar GCS injections improve arthritis. Systemic GCS use is recommended if it is required for enteropathic arthritis.

Sulfasalazine is used to treat UC and CD, and is effective in arthritis in SpA as well, however it does not improve axial symptoms.

TNF-blocking agents are very effective in resistant CD. Monoclonal antibodies targeting TNF are effective for treatment of both gut symptoms and arthritis.

The SAPHO (Synovitis, Acne, Pustulosis, Hyperostosis, Osteitis) syndrome is sometimes associated with pustulosis, acne form, skin rash associated with synovitis of the anterior chest wall and sacroiliac joints, spondylodiscitis, enthesopathy, aseptic osteomyelitis and hyperostosis.

The treatment is similar to SpA.

REFERENCES

[1]   Calin A, Porta J, Fries JF, Schurman DJ. Clinical history as a screening test for ankylosing spondylitis. JAMA 1977; 237(24): 2613-4.
[http://dx.doi.org/10.1001/jama.1977.03270510035017] [PMID: 140252]

[2]   Rudwaleit M, Metter A, Listing J, Sieper J, Braun J. Inflammatory back pain in ankylosing spondylitis: a reassessment of the clinical history for application as classification and diagnostic criteria. Arthritis Rheum 2006; 54(2): 569-78.
[http://dx.doi.org/10.1002/art.21619] [PMID: 16447233]

[3]   Sieper J, Rudwaleit M, Baraliakos X, *et al.* The Assessment of SpondyloArthritis international Society (ASAS) handbook: a guide to assess spondyloarthritis. Ann Rheum Dis 2009; 68 (Suppl. 2): 1-44.

[http://dx.doi.org/10.1136/ard.2008.104018] [PMID: 19433414]

[4]   Reveille JD, Sims AM, Danoy P, *et al.* Australo-Anglo-American Spondyloarthritis Consortium (TASC). Genome-wide association study of ankylosing spondylitis identifies non-MHC susceptibility loci. Nat Genet 2010; 42(2): 123-7.
[http://dx.doi.org/10.1038/ng.513] [PMID: 20062062]

[5]   van der Linden S, Valkenburg HA, Cats A. Evaluation of diagnostic criteria for ankylosing spondylitis. A proposal for modification of the New York criteria. Arthritis Rheum 1984; 27(4): 361-8.
[http://dx.doi.org/10.1002/art.1780270401] [PMID: 6231933]

[6]   Dougados M, van der Linden S, Juhlin R, *et al.* The European Spondylarthropathy Study Group preliminary criteria for the classification of spondylarthropathy. Arthritis Rheum 1991; 34(10): 1218-27.
[http://dx.doi.org/10.1002/art.1780341003] [PMID: 1930310]

[7]   Amor B, Dougados M, Listrat V, *et al.* [Evaluation of the Amor criteria for spondylarthropathies and European Spondylarthropathy Study Group (ESSG). A cross-sectional analysis of 2,228 patients]. Ann Med Interne (Paris) 1991; 142(2): 85-9.
[PMID: 2064170]

[8]   Rudwaleit M, van der Heijde D, Landewé R, *et al.* The development of Assessment of SpondyloArthritis international Society classification criteria for axial spondyloarthritis (part II): validation and final selection. Ann Rheum Dis 2009; 68(6): 777-83.
[http://dx.doi.org/10.1136/ard.2009.108233] [PMID: 19297344]

[9]   Rudwaleit M, van der Heijde D, Landewé R, *et al.* The Assessment of SpondyloArthritis International Society classification criteria for peripheral spondyloarthritis and for spondyloarthritis in general. Ann Rheum Dis 2011; 70(1): 25-31.
[http://dx.doi.org/10.1136/ard.2010.133645] [PMID: 21109520]

[10]   Garrett S, Jenkinson T, Kennedy LG, Whitelock H, Gaisford P, Calin A. A new approach to defining disease status in ankylosing spondylitis: the Bath Ankylosing Spondylitis Disease Activity Index. J Rheumatol 1994; 21(12): 2286-91.
[PMID: 7699630]

[11]   Lukas C, Landewé R, Sieper J, *et al.* Assessment of SpondyloArthritis international Society. Development of an ASAS-endorsed disease activity score (ASDAS) in patients with ankylosing spondylitis. Ann Rheum Dis 2009; 68(1): 18-24.
[http://dx.doi.org/10.1136/ard.2008.094870] [PMID: 18625618]

[12]   Calin A, Garrett S, Whitelock H, *et al.* A new approach to defining functional ability in ankylosing spondylitis: the development of the Bath Ankylosing Spondylitis Functional Index. J Rheumatol 1994; 21(12): 2281-5.
[PMID: 7699629]

[13]   Moncur C. Ankylosing Spondylitis Measures. The Ankylosing Spondylitis Quality of Life (ASQOL) Scale, Bath Ankylosing Spondylitis Disease Activity Index (BASDAI), Bath Ankylosing Spondylitis Functional Index (BASFI), Bath Ankylosing Spondylitis Global Score (BAS-G), Bath Ankylosing Spondylitis Metrology Index (BASMI), Dougados Functional Index (DFI), Health Assessment Questionnaire for the Spondyloarthropathies (HAQ-S), and Revised Leeds Disability Questionnaire (RLDQ). Arthritis Rheum 2003; 49: 197-209.
[http://dx.doi.org/10.1002/art.11412]

[14]   Rudwaleit M, Jurik AG, Hermann KG, *et al.* Defining active sacroiliitis on magnetic resonance imaging (MRI) for classification of axial spondyloarthritis: a consensual approach by the ASAS/OMERACT MRI group. Ann Rheum Dis 2009; 68(10): 1520-7.
[http://dx.doi.org/10.1136/ard.2009.110767] [PMID: 19454404]

[15]   van der Heijde D, Ramiro S, Landewé R, *et al.* 2016 update of the ASAS-EULAR management recommendations for axial spondyloarthritis. Ann Rheum Dis 2017; 76(6): 978-91.

[http://dx.doi.org/10.1136/annrheumdis-2016-210770] [PMID: 28087505]

[16] Helliwell PS, Taylor WJ. Classification and diagnostic criteria for psoriatic arthritis. Ann Rheum Dis 2005; 64 (Suppl. 2): 3-8.
[http://dx.doi.org/10.1136/ard.2004.032318] [PMID: 15708931]

[17] Feldman SR, Fleischer AB Jr, Reboussin DM, *et al.* The self-administered psoriasis area and severity index is valid and reliable. J Invest Dermatol 1996; 106(1): 183-6.
[http://dx.doi.org/10.1111/1523-1747.ep12329912] [PMID: 8592072]

[18] Sandre MK, Rohekar S. Psoriatic arthritis and nail changes: exploring the relationship. Semin Arthritis Rheum 2014; 44(2): 162-9.
[http://dx.doi.org/10.1016/j.semarthrit.2014.05.002] [PMID: 24932889]

[19] van der Heijde DM, van 't Hof M, van Riel PL, van de Putte LB. Development of a disease activity score based on judgment in clinical practice by rheumatologists. J Rheumatol 1993; 20(3): 579-81.
[PMID: 8478878]

[20] Heuft-Dorenbosch L, Spoorenberg A, van Tubergen A, *et al.* Assessment of enthesitis in ankylosing spondylitis. Ann Rheum Dis 2003; 62(2): 127-32.
[http://dx.doi.org/10.1136/ard.62.2.127] [PMID: 12525381]

[21] Ramiro S, Smolen JS, Landewé R, *et al.* Pharmacological treatment of psoriatic arthritis: a systematic literature review for the 2015 update of the EULAR recommendations for the management of psoriatic arthritis. Ann Rheum Dis 2016; 75(3): 490-8.
[http://dx.doi.org/10.1136/annrheumdis-2015-208466] [PMID: 26660203]

CHAPTER 3

Juvenile Idiopathic Arthritis and Acute Rheumatic Fever

Abstract: Juvenile Idiopathic Arthritis (JIA) is a group of diseases that starts before the age of 16 and is characterized by arthritis of at least one joint, lasting for more than 6 weeks and the origin of which is unknown. Symptoms of JIA include fever, rash, weakness, non-specific musculoskeletal pain and morning stiffness. Classification of JIA is based on symptoms that present during the first 6 months of the disease. Categories of JIA: systemic arthritis, oligoarthritis, a/persistent oligoarthritis b/extended oligoarthritis, polyarthritis (rheumatoid factor negative), polyarthritis (rheumatoid factor positive), psoriatic arthritis, enthesitis-related arthritis, undifferentiated arthritis.

There are no serological markers which may indicate JIA at diagnosis, therefore it is important to exclude other conditions which may mimick arthritis.

Initial treatment of children with arthritis begins with NSAIDs, intra-articular GCS and if these prove ineffective, methotraxate is used. Sulfasalazine, hydroxychloroquine or ciclosporin A may also be used. Biological therapies such as anti-TNFα, anti – IL1, IL6 blockade, abatacept show better improvement when they are added to methotrexate.

Acute rheumatic fever is a systemic inflammatory disease which occurs 2-3 weeks after infection with group A β-hemolytic streptococci. The acute form is characterized by: fever, arthritis, which is usually migratory and affects predominantly large joints. Cardiac manifestations due to involvement of the pericardium, myocardium, endocardium and heart valves may also occur. Neurological involvement is in the form of Sydenham's chorea.

Bed rest and antimicrobial therapy with penicillin is essential. Salicylate doses of 4 g may be required in adults. GCS is used in patients with severe carditis.

Keywords: Acute rheumatic fever, Anti-TNFα, Ciclosporin A, Endocarditis, Enthesitis-related arthritis, GCS, Group A β-hemolytic streptococci, Hydroxychloroquine, Juvenile Idiopathic Arthritis (JIA), Methotraxate, NSAIDs, Oligoarthritis, Penicillin, Polyarthritis, Psoriatic arthritis, Salicylate, Sulfasalazine, Systemic arthritis, Undifferentiated arthritis.

Małgorzata Wisłowska
All rights reserved-© 2018 Bentham Science Publishers

JUVENILE IDIOPATHIC ARTHRITIS

Introduction

Juvenile Idiopathic Arthritis (JIA) is a group of diseases that starts before 16 years of age and is characterized by arthritis of at least one joint that lasts for more than 6 weeks and of which the origin is unknown. The inflammatory process is caused by inflammatory cells infiltrating the joint and interacting with synovial fibroblasts, leading to a chronic inflammatory process in the synovial membrane and secreting synovial fluid.

The prevalence of JIA is around 1 in a 1000 and the incidence is approximately one in 10 000 children under the age of 16 years [1].

Differential diagnoses of JIA is important as arthritis in a child may be present in other diseases which are more common than JIA itself. There are no serological markers which may indicate JIA at diagnosis, therefore it is important to exclude other conditions associated with or mimicking arthritis.

Differential Diagnosis of Juvenile Idiopathic Arthritis when a Single Inflamed Joint is Involve:

Septic arthritis and osteomyelitis

Lyme disease

Reactive arthritis

Haemarthrosis secondary to trauma

Malignancy

Trauma

Differential Diagnosis of Juvenile Idiopathic Arthritis when more than one Inflamed Joints are Involve:

Systemic lupus erythematosus (SLE)

Juvenile dermatomyositis

Sarcoidosis

Sjögren syndrome

Mixed connective tissue disease (MCTD)

Henoch-Schenlein purpura

Reactive arthritis

Lyme disease

Malignancy

Immunodeficiency-associated arthritis

Inflammatory bowel disease-associated arthritis

Multifocal osteomyelitis

Cryopyrin-accociated periodic syndromes (CAPS)

Familial Mediterranean fever

Differential Diagnosis of Juvenile Idiopathic Arthritis when there are Systemic Features

Connective tissue diseases: SLE, MCTD, Kawasaki disease, other systemic vasculitis syndromes

Neoplasia

Infection

Inflammatory bowel disease

Familial Mediterranean fever, hyper-IgD syndrome, CAPS including CINCA syndrome (CINCA/NOMID), tumor necrosis factor receptor associated syndromes (TRAPS) and pharyngitis fever arthritis periodic fever (PFAPA) are inflammatory disorders characterized by recurrent attacks of fever and arthralgia or arthritis that often includes abdominal pains and rash resulting in gene mutations and present from birth or at a very early age. Genetic tests are indicated if the clinical features are suggestive.

JIA is a term used by WHO and used internationally and has replaced all past nomenclatures, including juvenile rheumatoid arthritis and juvenile chronic arthritis. JIA is a diagnosis of exclusion that involves all forms of arthritis that begins before the age of 16 years, persists for more than 6 weeks and are of unknown origin [2].

Common symptoms of JIA include fever, rash, weakness, anorexia, non-specific musculoskeletal pain and morning stiffness. Classification of JIA is based on symptoms that present during the first 6 months of disease.

Categories of JIA [2]

1. Systemic arthritis

2. Oligoarthritis

a. persistent oligoarthritis

b. extended oligoarthritis.

3. Polyarthritis (rheumatoid factor negative)

4. Polyarthritis (rheumatoid factor positive)

5. Psoriatic arthritis

6. Enthesitis-related arthritis

7. Undifferentiated arthritis.

Damage to the joint in JIA is due to the inflammatory process in joints as well as due to muscle atrophy. Discrepancy in leg length is due to involvement of a single knee joint. Local growth disturbances occur in places of inflammation, overgrowth which may be a result of inflammation, increased vascularization or undergrowth secondary to growth centre damage of epiphyseal plates of the juxtra-articular bone of the limb. Micrognathia and developmental anomalies of the hips may also occur.

Clinical Patterns of JIA

Systemic Arthritis or Still's Disease is characterized by a high spiking fever with systemic features such as a migratory, erythematous rash, generalized lymphadenopathy, serositis, myalgias, hepatosplenomegaly and abdominal pain. During fever peaks myalgia may be present. Leukocytosis (with neutrophilia), severe microcytic anaemia, thrombocytosis, high ESR and CRP concentration, hyperferritinaemia, and positive D-dimers or fibrin split products are very characteristic laboratory findings. Arthritis may include from one to many joints. Arthritis has a worst prognosis, with erosions, loss of joint motion, and severe growth delay. Macrophage activation syndrome is a severe complication of systemic arthritis and has a 10-15% mortality rate.

Macrophage activation syndrome (MAS) is a reactive hemophagocytic lymphohistiocytosis characterised by fever, pancytopenia, hepatomegaly, liver insufficiency, a coagulopathy with haemorrhagic and neurological manifestations. Elevated transaminases and triglycerides and increased ferritin concentrations are very characteristic. Phagocytosis of haemopoietic cells by macrophages in bone marrow may be found. Macrophages express CD163, a scavenger receptor that recognizes haptoglobin-hemoglobin complexes. These complexes within the macrophages results in production of ferritin, which explains hyperferritinemia.

MAS may also be observed in patients with polyarthritis. It occurs in around 7% of patients with systemic JIA. Fibrin degradation products are present in MAS and hypofibrinogenaemia is induced by diffused intravascular coagulation. Active phagocytosis by macrophages and histiocytes may be observed on bone marrow examination. MAS must be treated rapidly with intravenous methylprednisolone pulse therapy and ciclosporin. Early recognition of the syndrome results in complete resolution. It reverses rapid deterioration and disseminated intravascular coagulopathy (DIC). Etoposide is added in some patients with relapsing disease.

JIA is a polygenic inflammatory disease that activates of the innate immune system [3]. Sensitivity to interleukin 1 blockade may explain this characteristic heterogenicity [4]. The disease may be monocyclic or is characterized by relapses followed by intervals of remission in half of patients. The long-term prognosis of these patients is usually good. The disease may be unremitting in the other half of patients with chronic arthritis.

Systemic onset JIA encompasses approximately 10% of cases of arthritis that begin in childhood [4].

Oligoarthritis is an arthritis that targets four joints or fever during the first 6 months of disease in the absence of features (psoriasis, RF positivity, high spiking fever). Common features are asymmetrical arthritis, an early onset (before 6 years of age), a female predominance, positive antinuclear antibodies and a high risk for developing chronic iridocyclitis and consistent human leucocyte antigen (HLA) associations (HLA-DRB1*08). Oligoarthritis represents up to 50% of all JIA cases.

The International League of Association for Rheumatology (ILAR) [2] classification include two categories: persistent oligoarthritis, in which the disease involves four joints or less, and extended oligoarthritis, in which arthritis extended to more than four joints after the first 6 months of disease. It has been shown that ANA-positive patients with persistent or with extended oligoarthritis have the same symptoms. Predictors of the extended phenotype is upper limb involvement and a high ESR at onset. Children with persistent oligoarthritis, which may occur in up to 50% of patients have good articular outcome.

Oligoarthritis is predominantly a disease of the lower limbs, with the involvement of knee joint. The next localization are the ankles. In about 30-50% of cases a single joint is involved. Acute phase reactants are normal or slightly increased.

In around one-third of patients chronic nongranulomatous anterior uveitis develops and involves the iris and the ciliary body (iridocyclitis) and may cause severe visual impairment. This uveitis is asymptomatic. Unilateral or bilateral ocular involvement may be observed. In most cases it occurs at the time of diagnosis, however in a hand-fill of patients (<10%) it may precede the onset of arthritis. Most children develop iridocyclitis within 5-7 years after onset of arthritis. The course of iridocyclitis may be relapsing or chronic and does not parallel the course of the arthritis. Children with iridocyclitis may develope complications, including posterior synechiae, band keratopathy, cataract and glaucoma. The outcome of iridocyclitis depends on early diagnosis and treatment, however because iridocyclitis is asymptomatic at onset, screening children with oligoarthritis every 3 months by slip-lamp examination is mandatory.

Polyarthritis (RF Negative) is an arthritis that affects five or more joints during the first 6 months of disease in the absence of RF. It occurs in 15-20% of JIA cases. Two clinical phenotypes are present.

The first form of disease is characterized by symmetrical synovitis of big and small joints, onset at school age, raised ESR, negative ANAs and variable outcomes. This may be similar to adult-onset RF-negative rheumatoid arthritis.

The second form is similar to ANA-positive, early-onset oligoarthritis and involve a female predominance, increased incidence of chronic iridocyclitis and association with HLA-DRB1*08. Similarities between the second subset and ANA-positive, early-onset oligoarthritis may suggest that they are the same disease. The long-term prognosis of ANA-positive, early-onset, RF-negative polyarthritis is worse than that of persistent oligoarthritis and similar to that of extended oligoarthritis. ANA-positive patients must have slit-lamp examinations every 3 months due to an increased risk of chronic iridocyclitis.

Polyarthritis (RF Positive) is the same as in adult RA in features and prognosis. It primarily affects girls, and presents in late childhood or adolescence. It progresses rapidly and is destructive, with rheumatoid nodules. RF is positive and antibodies to cyclic citrullinated peptides (CCP) are found. It affects less than 5% of patients with JIA.

Psoriatic Arthritis is an arthritis with a psoriatic rash or, if the rash is absent, the presence of arthritis and any of the following: family history of psoriasis in a first-degree relative, dactylitis (swelling of one or more digits and nail pitting). Arthritis may occur before skin psoriasis many years before and is not required for diagnosis in a child. Articular involvement in psoriatic arthritis is often asymmetrical, and may affect both small and large joints such as oligoarthritis. Diagnosis is confirmed by a family history of a first-degree relative with psoriasis. Asymptomatic uveitis occurs with the same risk of blindness as in oligoarthritis.

Psoriatic arthritis occurs in 5-10% of all JIA cases. Two groups of patients may be identified:

1. First group with features, as in adult psoriatic arthritis, or spondyloarthritis.

2. Second group that involves features such as early age onset, ANA positivity, asymmetrical arthritis, female predominance, increased incidence of chronic iridocyclitis of ANA-positive, early-onset oligoarthritis. ANA-positive patients have to be checked every 3 months by slit-lamp examination.

Enthesitis-related Arthritis is undifferentiated spondyloarthritis. It begins after the age of 6 years and affects boys more often than girls. It is characterized by lower limb arthritis complicated by enthesitis of the plantar fascia, the insertion of the Achilles tendon into the calcaneum, and around and below the patella. It may lead to ankylosing spondylitis in the future. Symptoms of sacroiliitis and spinal arthritis are uncommon. Uveitis affects these patients and is symptomatic, with red eyes, photophobia and pain. A family history is often positive and HLA-B27 antigen may be found in 50% of patients, while ANA is negative. Hip involvement is frequent.

Enthesitis-related arthritis accounts for about 5-10% of JIA cases.

Undifferentiated Arthritis is a disease which does not fulfill inclusion criteria for any category, or fulfill the criteria for more than one category. There are a large number of combinations of classification criteria which are needed for the disease to be placed in the undifferentiated arthritis category. The most commonly observed combination of features is oligoarthritis and psoriatic arthritis, and a positive family history for psoriasis in the absence of other criteria to fulfil the definition of psoriatic arthritis. Other common patterns include a positive family history for either psoriasis or HLA-B27 related diseases in combination with polyarthritis and, less commonly, systemic arthritis. The presence of a positive RF test without polyarthritis may be another combination of the undifferentiated arthritis. About 10 -15% of all JIA cases are included in this category.

Variations in Skeletal Development

Children do not grow in a linear fashion, including skeletal alignment or growth velocity. Asymmetry, often minor, may be present on physical examination. This includes foot sizes, as well as in the size and length of legs. Although these changes do not need attention, changes in skeletal alignment such as knock knees (genu valgum) and bow legs (genu varum) often cause parental concern.

Infants are born with a physiological varus knee angle which gradually straightens with age to neutral alignment between 18 months and 2 years of age. Further normal growth results in changes in knee alignment to a valgus position which peaks between 5 and 7 years of age (up to 15 years), resulting in an intermalleolar distance at the ankles of up to 5 cm. Therefore it is normal to observe varying degrees of knee varus (bow legs) or valgus (knock knee) and it is common, and no intervention is required.

Children with JIA may develop increasing knee valgus due to differential overgrowth of the medial femoral condyle as a consequence of the inflammatory process. If the intermalleolar distance reaches beyond 10 cm, surgical intervention may be necessary.

A medial longitudinal foot arch, or a stable hindfoot position is not observed in infants at birth. Therefore, a marked angle valgus and a "flat foot" (pes planus) is observed, which is obvious once the infant begins to walk. Children are more flexible than adults, and the range of normal joint movement in children is greater. However if it reaches beyond this range, this is due to the skeletal malalignment and increased muscle tension is required to maintain posture which results in joint and muscle pain.

DIAGNOSIS

It is important to exclude differential diagnoses in child with clinical features of musculoskeletal pain. We can use imaging diagnosis like as radiographs of joints to exclude fractures, avascular necrosis, periostitis, osteomyelitis, bone neoplasia and bone dysplasia. Ultrasound of the hip joints can show effusion. MRI shows the anatomical changes in the musculoskeletal system.

Imaging studies are the most useful investigative tests. Plain radiographs, ultrasonography, and MRI are useful in excluding other diseases. Synovial biopsy does not confirm diagnose of JIA, but it is useful in excluding neoplasia, sarcoidosis or pigmented villonodular synovitis.

Plain X-ray radiographs have a role in excluding fractures, avascular necrosis of bone, bone neoplasia, bone dysplasia, osteomyelitis, slipped upper femoral epiphysis and Scheuermann disease, It is also important in assessing disease progression.

Ultrasonography of joints shows joint effusion in the hip and other joints which cannot be examined by physical examination.

MRI (with Gadolinum contrast) of joints confirms the presence of early synovial inflammation and early erosions.

The interpretation of imaging is different in adults because the skeleton is undergoing its development and mineralization.

No diagnostic tests exist to diagnose JIA. RF and ANAs may be used to subclassify JIA. RF is used to subclassify children with polyarthritis, and ANAs are used to determine the risk of chronic anterior uveitis and to identify an early-onset arthritis. HLA B27 may be present in some of the JIA patients.

Tests for acute phase reactants (ESR and CRP) may be useful for monitoring disease activity.

The blood count is useful to diagnose neoplastic causes of cytopenia. Neutrophilic leukocytosis, thrombocytosis and microcytic anaemia are common in systemic JIA. A sudden drop of leukocyte count and platelets occurs during MAS.

The ESR is raised in systemic arthritis in about one-third of patients with JIA.

CRP is normal in up to half of patients with JIA.

A sudden increase of transaminases in systemic JIA occurs during MAS.

ANA positivity in JIA suggests a higher risk of developing iridocyclitis and requires a slit-lamp examination every 3 months.

Microbiology diagnosis excludes infectious diseases such as Lyme disease or brucellosis, tuberculosis, viral infections, enteric bacterial pathogens or acute rheumatic fever (elevated ASO titers). Synovial fluid analysis is important to exclude septic arthritis.

Blood cultures should also be obtained.

Urine analysis and urine catecholamines should be checked to exclude renal involvement in other autoimmune diseases or neuroblastoma.

TREATMENT

Early diagnosis, patient and family disease education, aggressive medical treatment and physical interventions are very important. A multidisciplinary team, consisting of physiotherapists, occupational therapists, social workers, psychologists, nutritionists, ophthalmologists (detection and monitoring of uveitis), orthopaedic surgeons, dentists and orthotists/podiatrists should provide care for the patient.

Initial treatment of children with arthritis starts with NSAIDs and intra-articular GCS and if these prove ineffective, methotraxate is used. Sulfasalazine, hydroxychloroquine or ciclosporin A may also be used. Biological therapies such as anti-TNFα, anti – IL1 and IL6 blockade and abatacept show better improvement when they are add to methotrexate.

Treatment of JIA cause suppression of inflammation, decrease in pain and prevention of joint destruction. Pain is associated with inflammation and joint destruction and affects the child's quality of life. NSAIDs are continued for 4-8 weeks before changes to treatment are made. Adverse effects include abdominal pain and are minimized by taking NSAID with food. Rarely bronchospasm may occur (mild asthma is not a contraindication in the use of NSAIDs in children). Naproxen has the additional risk of inducing pseudo-porphyria. Salicylates have been replaced by NSAIDs in paediatric practice because of the association of aspirin with Reye syndrome. The majority of patients with early JIA do not respond completely to NSAIDs and need more aggressive treatment.

Glucocorticosteroids (GCS)

Intra-articular GCS are frequently used in JIA. A single injection improves signs of inflammation for several months. Chronic use of systemic steroids should be avoided if possible because of adverse effects such as growth and immune suppression, cataract, diabetes, necrosis of bone, vertebral fractures and Cushing syndrome. However, in cases of aggressive inflammatory disease, pulses of intravenous methylprednisolone may help to control devastating arthritis and may be life-saving in pericarditis with tamponade or rapidly progressive MAS. The use of oral prednisolone is limited to a short time and low dose.

Chronic inflammation affects linear growth but growth retardation is secondary to prolonged steroid therapy. One of the side effects of steroid therapy is the inhibition of growth.

DISEASE-MODIFYING ANTIRHEUMATIC DRUGS

After 4-12 weeks, disease-modifying antirheumatic drugs (DMARDs) such as methotrexate may be introduced if signs of inflammation persist. Symptoms of arthritis improves in 70% of children with JIA.

Methotrexate initial dose is 10-15 mg/m^2/week. It is usually given orally 1 h before food to improve absorption. Subcutaneous methotrexate may be an alternative in some patients. Efficiency of methotrexate is observed after 1-3 months. The most common adverse events associated with methotrexate are nausea, abdominal pain, raised liver enzymes, and rarely, hair loss and bone marrow suppression. Children taking methotrexate must have monthly blood monitoring to observe abdominal liver function and bone marrow suppression. Oral folate supplements may limit side effects.

Leflunomide has the same efficiency as methotrexate and can be an alternative drug.

Sulfasalazine has been efficacious in oligoarthritis and polyarthritis, particularly effective in early rheumatoid arthritis. It is well tolerated, but sometimes has dermatological adverse events and rarely aplastic anaemia. The dosage of 30-50 mg/kg/day is divided into three doses.

A soluble tumor necrosis factor alpha receptors and monoclonal antibodies against TNF alpha, may be started in children with long-term disability due to the duration and destruction of inflammatory synovitis. The use of these drugs has added a new option in the treatment of potentially disabling arthritis in both adults and children and the resulting outcomes have significantly altered the natural history and stopped the progression of disease in a substantial proportion of patients.

The soluble TNFalpha receptor, etanercept, is approved for the treatment of children with polyarthritis/extended oligoarthritis whose disease is not adequately controlled with methotrexate or who are intolerant to it [5]. A large multicenter trial showed that children with severe, methotrexate-resistant polyarthritis showed clinical improvement with more than 2 years of continuous etanercept treatment [5]. Etanercept was well tolerated and there were no adverse events. Regular (1-2 month) monitoring of blood counts and chemistry studies are recommended.

Etanercept should be stopped in the event of fever or other signs of significant infection. Long-term follow-up registries for use of etanercept in JIA show tolerable side effects [6].

Adalimumab, a fully humanized monoclonal antibody to TNFalpha, showed a good efficacy in children with polyarticular JIA in combination with methotrexate. Adalimumab seems to be efficient for treatment of JIA-associated uveitis. Patients treated with adalimumab rarely have side effects such as infections, elevation of transaminases, hyperlipidaemia or pancytopenia.

Infliximab is a chimera monoclonal antibody against TNF alpha. It is effective in RA but is not used in JIA. Infusion reactions are common [7].

Anti-TNFalpha therapy should be stopped if fever or other signs of infection occurs. Active tuberculosis must be excluded before starting TNFalpha blocking agents.

Golimumab another TNFalpha antibody is approved for the treatment of children with a body mass more than 40 kg.

Anakinra (IL-1 receptor antagonist) and canakinumab (anti-IL-1beta antibody) are effective in patients with systemic JIA. Anakinra is very effective in controlling fever and rash in systemic JIA.

Tocilizumab (anti-IL-6) is another option for treatment of JIA [8]. It is effective in severe, persistent systemic JIA [9]. Adverse events include infections, neutropenia, and increased aminotransferase levels. Serious adverse events may be anaphylactic reaction, gastrointestinal haemorrhage, bronchitis and gastroenteritis.

Abatacept (CTLA-4 Ig), an inhibitor of costimulatory signals during antigen presentation, is good option for patients with polyarthritis who are resistant to conventional treatment.

Ciclosporin A has been used to control treatment-resistant arthritis. It has also been combined with methotrexate to treat uveitis. Side effects include gingivalis hyperplasia and hirsutism. In chronic use, ciclosporin A gives hypertension and progressive renal disease. It is very useful in treating MAS with high-dose of intravenous methylprednisolone.

Cyclophosphamide is a disease-modifying antirheumatic drug also used to treat cancer. It is rarely considered, however, it may be used in patients unresponsive to all other available treatments.

Autologous stem cell transplantation is procedure very rarely use in children in extreme disease.

COMPLICATION OF JIA

Complications in JIA patients are MAS, chronic anterior uveitis, growth disturbances, cardiac disease, secondary amyloidosis, osteoporosis.

Chronic anterior uveitis is the most important complication of oligoarthritis associated with ANA (+) disease; however, it may occur in other forms of JIA as well. Routine examination of the eye every 3 months for ANA (+) oligoarthritis JIA is recommended in order to avoid blindness.

Growth disturbance is the major problem for children with arthritis. Biological treatment and the decreased use of corticosteroids have reduced this complication.

Pericarditis, myocarditis and endocarditis are rare complications in JIA.

Osteoporosis may also occur in polyarticular JIA.

Infections are serious complications in an immunosuppressed child. Vaccinations should be applied.

The majority of deaths in JIA were related to amyloidosis. The rate of this complication has markedly decreased with improved treatment.

PROGNOSIS OF JIA

At least one-third of children with JIA will continue to have active arthritis into their adult years and will need to participate in adult healthcare services, usually in rheumatology clinics [10, 11].

ACUTE RHEUMATIC FEVER

This is a systemic inflammatory disease which occurs 2-3 weeks after infection with group A β-hemolytic streptococci. The disease is mediated by an autoimmune response to antigenic components of the organism that cross-react with similar epitopes in human tissues such as the heart, joints, brain and skin.

CLINICAL FEATURES

The acute form of the illness is characterized by: fever, arthritis, which is usually migratory and affects predominantly the large joints. Cardiac manifestations due to involvement of the pericardium, myocardium, endocardium and heart valves. Neurological involvement which manifests as Sydenham's chorea. Cutaneous involvement consisting of erythema marginatum and subcutaneous nodules which are less common.

EPIDEMIOLOGY

Acute rheumatic fever was common in Europe and North America at the beginning of the 20th century. Since then there has been a rapid decline in the incidence of the disease and this was further accelerated with the introduction of antibiotics in 1950.

JONES CRITERIA, updated 1992 [12].

Major Manifestations: I. carditis, II. polyarthritis, III. chorea, IV. erythema marginatum, V. subcutaneous nodules.

Minor Manifestations: I. arthralgia, II. fever, III. laboratory findings: elevated acute phase reactants, erythrocyte sedimentation rate, CRP and prolonged P – R interval.

Supporting evidence of antecedent group A streptococcal infection in the last 45 days: positive throat culture or rapid streptococcal infection test, elevated or rising streptococcal antibody titer or recent scarlet fever.

If supported by evidence of preceding group A streptococcal infection, the presence of two major manifestations or of one major and two minor manifestations indicates a high probability of acute rheumatic fever.

In the revised 2015 Jones criteria, a low, medium and high-risk population was identified. A low risk population is one in which cases of acute rheumatic fever occur in <=2/100 000 school-age children or rheumatic heart disease is diagnosed in <=1/1000 patients at any age during one year.

DIAGNOSTIC CRITERIA FOR RHEUMATIC FEVER – modified 2015 Jones criteria [13].

MAJOR CRITERIA

Low risk population	High risk population
Carditis (clinical or subclinical)	Carditis (clinical or subclinical)
Arthritis – only polyarthritis	Arthritis – monoarthritis or polyarthritis
Chorea	Polyarthralgia
Erythema marginatum	Chorea
Subculaneous nodules	Erythema marginatum
	Subcutaneous nodules

MINOR CRITERIA

Low risk population	High risk population
Polyarthralgia	Monoarthralgia
Hyperpyrexia (≥38.5 ° C)	Hyperpyrexia (≥38.0 °C)
ESR ≥60 mm/h and/or CRP ≥3.0 mg/dl	ESR ≥30 mm/h and/or CRP ≥3 mg/dl
Prolonged PR interval if there is no carditis as a major criteria	Prolonged PR interval if there is no carditis as a major criteria

The diagnosis of rheumatic fever in the whole population with evidence of astecendent group A beta-hemolytic streptococcal infection requires a confirmation of two major criteria or one major and two minor criteria – the first episode of the disease.

The diagnosis of subsequent episodes of the disease requires a confirmation of two major criteria or one major and two minor criteria or three minor criteria [13].

TREATMENT

Bed rest and antimicrobial therapy – adequate treatment of the streptococcal pharyngeal infection is essential to avoid prolonged and repetitive exposure to streptococcal antigen. The drug of choice is still phenoxymethylpenicillin orally at the following doses: adults and chidren with a body weight >40 kg – 2-3 MIU/day in 2 divided doses every 12 hours for 10 days, children with a body weight < 40 kg – 100,000 to 200,000 IU/kg/day in 2 divided doses every 12 hours for 10 days.

Benzylpenicillin, administered intramuscularly at a single dose (only in hospital settings), is acceptable, for adults and children with a body weight > 40 kg – 1.2 MIU, children with a body weight < 40 kg – 600,000 IU.

In patient with hypersensitivity to penicillin (except for immediate-type reactions), first generation cephalosporins (cefadroxil or cephalexin) are used.

Cefadroxil: adults and children with a body weight > 40 kg – 1 g, children with a body weight < 40 kg – 30 mg/kg, in a single dose for 10 days

Cefalexin: adult 500 mg twice per day, children 25-50 mg/kg/day in 2 doses for 10 days.

Macrolides should only be administered in patients with immediate-type hypersensitivity to beta-lactam antibiotics. The following can be used: erythromycin, clarithromycin and azithromycin.

Erythromycin: adults and children with a body weight > 40 kg – 0.2-0.4 g every 6-8 hours, children with a body weight < 40 kg – 30-50 mg/kg/day in 3-4 doses, for 10 days.

Clarithromycin: adults and children with a body weight > 40 kg – 250-500 mg every 12 hours, children with a body weight < 40 kg – 15 mg/kg/day in 2 doses, for 10 days.

Azithromycin: adults and children with a body weight > 40 kg – 500 mg on the first day, then 250 mg for three consecutive days, children with a body weight < 40 kg – a single daily dose of 12 mg/kg/day for 5 days or 20 mg/kg/day for 3 days

Secondary prevention of subsequent rheumatic fever relapses through the chronic anti-streptococcal treatment should be administered from 5 to 10 years from the last rheumatic fever relapse, or up to 21 years of age.

In rheumatic fever cases with carditis leading to chronic valvular heart disease the prevention should be administered for 10 years or until 40 years of age.

Secondary prevention makes use of benzathine benzylpenicillin, intramuscularly: in adults and children with a body weight > 20 kg – 1.2 MIU, in children with a body weight < 20 kg – 600,000 IU every 4 weeks.

Phenoxymerhylpenicillin is administered orally at a dose 2 x 250 mg *i.e.* 2 x 400,000 IU).

In the case of heart involvement, GCS are used prednisone at a dose 1-2mg/kg/day for 2-3 weeks, then the dose should be reduced gradually. The total duration of GCS treatment is 6 weeks. During the period of prednisone dose reduction, acetylsalicylic acid should be initiated – at 60 mg/kg/day.

The treatment of chorea is based on sedatives, antiepileptics, in some cases GCS, immunoglobulins or plasmapheresis.

REFERENCES

[1]   Prakken B, Albani S, Martini A. Juvenile idiopathic arthritis. Lancet 2011; 377(9783): 2138-49.
        [http://dx.doi.org/10.1016/S0140-6736(11)60244-4] [PMID: 21684384]

[2]   Petty RE, Southwood TR, Manners P, *et al.* International League of Associations for Rheumatology classification of juvenile idiopathic arthritis: second revision, Edmonton, 2001. J Rheumatol 2004; 31(2): 390-2.
        [PMID: 14760812]

[3]   Mellins ED, Macaubas C, Grom AA. Pathogenesis of systemic juvenile idiopathic arthritis: some answers, more questions. Nat Rev Rheumatol 2011; 7(7): 416-26.
        [http://dx.doi.org/10.1038/nrrheum.2011.68] [PMID: 21647204]

[4]   Pascual V, Allantaz F, Arce E, Punaro M, Banchereau J. Role of interleukin-1 (IL-1) in the pathogenesis of systemic onset juvenile idiopathic arthritis and clinical response to IL-1 blockade. J Exp Med 2005; 201(9): 1479-86.
[http://dx.doi.org/10.1084/jem.20050473] [PMID: 15851489]

[5]   Lovell DJ, Ruperto N, Giannini EH, Martini A. Advances from clinical trials in juvenile idiopathic arthritis. Nat Rev Rheumatol 2013; 9(9): 557-63.
[http://dx.doi.org/10.1038/nrrheum.2013.105] [PMID: 23838613]

[6]   Shakoor N, Michalska M, Harris CA, Block JA. Drug-induced systemic lupus erythematosus associated with etanercept therapy. Lancet 2002; 359(9306): 579-80.
[http://dx.doi.org/10.1016/S0140-6736(02)07714-0] [PMID: 11867114]

[7]   Ruperto N, Lovell DJ, Cuttica R, *et al.* A randomized, placebo-controlled trial of infliximab plus methotrexate for the treatment of polyarticular-course juvenile rheumatoid arthritis. Arthritis Rheum 2007; 56(9): 3096-106.
[http://dx.doi.org/10.1002/art.22838] [PMID: 17763439]

[8]   Herlin T. Tocilizumab: The evidence for its place in the treatment of juvenile idiopathic arthritis. Core Evid 2010; 4: 181-9.
[PMID: 20694074]

[9]   Woo P, Wilkinson N, Prieur AM, *et al.* Open label phase II trial of single, ascending doses of MRA in Caucasian children with severe systemic juvenile idiopathic arthritis: proof of principle of the efficacy of IL-6 receptor blockade in this type of arthritis and demonstration of prolonged clinical improvement. Arthritis Res Ther 2005; 7(6): R1281-8.
[http://dx.doi.org/10.1186/ar1826] [PMID: 16277681]

[10]   Foster HE, Marshall N, Myers A, Dunkley P, Griffiths ID. Outcome in adults with juvenile idiopathic arthritis: a quality of life study. Arthritis Rheum 2003; 48(3): 767-75.
[http://dx.doi.org/10.1002/art.10863] [PMID: 12632431]

[11]   Szer IS, Kimura Y, Malleson PN, *et al.* Arthritis in children and adolescents: juvenile idiopathic arthritis. UK: Oxford University Press 2006.

[12]   Dajani AS, Ajoub EM, Bierman FZ. Guidelines for the diagnosis of rheumatic fever: Jones Criteria, updated 1992. JAMA 1992; 87: 300-7.

[13]   Gewitz M, Baltimore R, Tani L. Revision of the Jones Criteria for the Diagnosis of Acute Rheumatic Fever in the Era of Doppler Echocardiography: A Scientific Statement From the American Heart Association. Circulation 2015; 131: 1806-1818.

CHAPTER 4

Systemic Lupus Erythematosus and Antiphospholipid Syndrome

Abstract: Systemic lupus erythematosus (SLE) is an inflammatory disease involving many systems, with different clinical features and laboratory findings. The etiology of SLE is unknown.

The pathogenesis of SLE may derive from genetic as well as environmental factors. Overproduction of autoantibodies causes cytotoxic damage and takes part in immune complex formation causing inflammation.

Clinical features may be general or result from inflammation in different organ systems including skin and mucous membranes, joints, kidneys, brain, serous membranes, lungs, heart and occasionally the gastrointestinal tract.

The morbidity and mortality is associated with the involvement of vital organs, especially the kidneys and central nervous system, and is due to direct tissue damage or as a result of therapy.

Lupus management is based on disease activity.

Antimalarial drugs are effective for acute and chronic lupus rashes. Most clinical symptoms of SLE respond to GCS, however the adverse effects of GCS cause an increase in morbidity and must be tapered and withdrawn. Severe lupus (*e.g.* proliferative lupus nephritis, CNS involvement or severe thrombocytopenia) is treated by pulse IV methylprednisolone (MP) followed by oral GCS (0.5 mg/kg/day) and MMF or IV CYC, followed by less toxic AZA, MMF.

To diagnose antiphospholipid syndrome (APS), a patient must have both a clinical event (thrombosis or pregnancy loss) and an antiphospholipid antibody (aPL), documented by a solid-phase serum assay (anticardiolipin – aCL), an inhibitor of phospholipid-dependent clotting (lupus anticoagulant – LA), or both.

APS is treated by anticoagulation such as warfarin, heparin, and low-molecular-weight heparin and often in association with low-dose aspirin.

Małgorzata Wisłowska

Keywords: ANA, Anticardiolipin, Anticoagulation, Antimalarials, Antiphospholipid antibody, Antiphospholipid syndrome, Autoantibody, AZA, CNS involvement, Complement deficiency, CYC, dsDNA, GCS, Low-molecular-weight heparin, Lupus anticoagulant, Lupus nephritis, MMF, Pregnancy loss, Systemic lupus erythematosus (SLE), Warfarin.

SYSTEMIC LUPUS ERYTHEMATOSUS

Introduction

Systemic lupus erythematosus (SLE) is an inflammatory disease, involving many systems, with different clinical features and laboratory findings. The etiology of SLE is unknown.

Epidemiology

The prevalence of SLE is around 20 to 50/100.000, and is more prevalent in women, during their reproductive years [1].

History

In 1872 Kaposi described the systemic nature of lupus.Before that, the term "lupus" latin meaning wolf, was used in the 18th century to describe different skin conditions. It was considered a chronic dermatological disorder for many decades.

ETIOLOGY AND PATHOGENESIS

The pathogenesis of SLE may be derived from genetic as well as environmental factors. Immunological tolerance dysfunction is observed, which is seen as abnormal immune responses against endogenous nuclear and other self-antigens [2]. Overproduction of autoantibodies causes cytotoxic damage and takes part in immune complex formation causing inflammation. Genes linked to immune response and inflammation, DNA repair, adherence of inflammatory cells to the endothelium and tissue response to injury play an important role, similar to Toll-like receptors and type 1 interferon signaling pathways [3]. The risk for SLE may be influenced by DNA methylation and post-translational histone modifications, which can be genetically determined or environmentally induced [4]. An epigenetic factor is DNA methylation, which plays a role in X chromosome inactivation [4]. SLE may be triggered by ultraviolet light, demethylating drugs, cosmetic products and infectious or endogenous viruses [5]. Different cells and molecules play a role in apoptosis, innate and adaptive immune responses and are involved in SLE pathogenesis. INFγ produced by apoptosis-related endogenous nucleic acids induce autoimmunity by breaking self-tolerance through activation of antigen-presenting cells. Immune complexes are cleared by Fc and complement receptors. Failure to clear immune complexes results in tissue deposition and tissue injury. Tissue damage is mediated by inflammatory cells, reactive oxygen intermediates, production of inflammatory cytokines and modulation of the coagulation cascade. DNA degradation, which results from mutation of TREX1, may activate the IFN-stimulatory DNA response and cause immune-mediated injury to the vasculature [6].

CLINICAL PICTURE

Clinical features may be general or result from inflammation in different organ systems including skin and mucous membranes, joints, kidneys, brain, serous membranes, lungs, heart and occasionally the gastrointestinal tract. Single or a combination of organ systems may be involved.

The morbidity and mortality is associated with the involvement of vital organs, especially the kidneys and central nervous system, and is due to direct tissue damage or as a result of therapy.

Mucocutaneous involvement is always present in SLE. The "butterfly" rash, which is pathognomonic, is an erythematous, raised lesion, with pruritis or pain, in malar distribution and exacerbated after exposure to sunlight. Discoid lesions are characterized by erythematous, infiltrated plaques covered by a scale that extends into dilated hair follicles on the face, neck and scalp, but also occur on the ears and on the upper body. They heal leaving depressed central scars, atrophy, teleangiectasias and depigmentation. Other rashes present in SLE is lupus profundus, seen as a firm nodular lesion and lupus tumidus, seen as photo-distributed lesions with chronic pink indurated plaques. Alopecia, which is severe hair loss, is associated with SLE.

Oral ulcers in SLE are usually painless.

Joint involvement is non-erosive, non-deforming and arthralgias/ arthritis affects the small joints of the hands, wrists and knees. Jacoub-type arthropathy is the deformation of the hands such as ulnar drift at the metacarpophalangeal joints, swan-neck and boutonniere deformity, and hyperextension at the interphalangeal joint of the thumb without erosions.

Myalgia and muscle tenderness are present and avascular necrosis of bone may be seen as well.

Renal involvement is a major cause of morbidity and occurs in 40-70% of patients [7]. Immune complex formation/deposition in the kidney results in intraglomerular inflammation and proliferation of renal cells. Proteinuria is the main feature in nephritis and therefore urinary analysis is important. Haematuria indicates glomerular or tubulointestinal disease and the erythrocytes are dysmorphic (fragmental or misshaped). Granular and fatty casts indicate proteinuric status and red blood cells, white blood cells and mixed cellular casts indicate nephritic states, while broad and waxy casts indicate chronic renal failure. In severe cases urine sediment contains cells and casts ("telescopic urine sediment") due to severe glomerular and tubular disease along with renal failure. Renal biopsy is the gold standard to diagnose lupus nephritis (LN) [7].

Central nervous system (CNS) and the peripheral nervous system are also involved in SLE. The ACR describes classification criteria for CNS and peripheral nervous system syndromes seen in SLE, which are known as neuropsychiatric SLE (NPSLE) syndromes [8].

NPSLE manifestations and the association between SLE and headache is controversial. Headaches are common but are not related to lupus, however they are sometimes involved in severe lupus and must be investigated, when they don't respond to analgesics and are accompanied by fever, altered mental status, and meningeal or focal neurological signs. Cognitive dysfunction occurs in 20-30% of patients with SLE but is mild [8]. Psychosis occurs in up to 3.5% and is characterized by delusions or hallucinations [8]. Seizures are more common and occur in 9-10% of cases. They may be associated with antiphospholipid antibodies [8]. Demyelination, transverse myelopathy and chorea are rare manifestations, each occurring in < 1% of patients [8].

Myelitis may present as upper motor neuron spasticity, hyper-reflexia or lower motor neurone syndrome with flaccid paralysis and decreased reflexes. This is associated with neuromyelitis optica (NMO) and the presence of antibodies to aquaporin (NMO-IgG) [9].

Cardiovascular features include pericarditis. They occur in 15-25% of patients with SLE. Pericardial effusions may be mild to moderate or asymptomatic. Myocardial involvement is rare, and may present with fever, dyspnoea, tachycardia and congestive heart failure. Features of left ventricular dysfunction, non-specific ST/T wave changes and decreased ejection fraction occurs in 80% of patients.

Cardiovascular diseases involve accelerated atherosclerosis and valvular heart disease and cause increased morbidity and mortality. Arteriosclerosis and valvular heart disease lead to myocardial infarction and stroke. Valvular heart disease associated with antiphospholipid syndrome secondary to SLE is common. Other common findings include diffuse thickening of the mitral and aortic valves followed by vegetations, valvular regurgitation and stenosis. Libman–Sacks vegetations with acute thrombus, healed vegetations with or without hyalinized thrombus, or both are pathological finding which may be found on examination.

SLE involves pleuritis, which is the most common pleuropulmonary manifestation in SLE. Pleural effusion was reported in up to 50% of patients. Effusions are usually bilateral and are exudative in nature with higher glucose and lower lactate dehydrogenase levels than those found in RA.

Interstitial lung disease occurs in 3-12% of SLE patients but it is not severe. Pneumonitis (cough, dyspnoea, pleuritis pain, hypoxemia and fever) occurs in 1-4%. Pulmonary haemorrhage is a rare complication of SLE but is usually fatal when present.

The "shrinking lung syndrome", secondary to diaphragmatic dysfunction, is characterized by progressive dyspnoea and small lung capacities on chest X-rays. Pulmonary hypertension may be a complication of SLE and is life-threatening.

Lymphadenopathy occurs in about 40% of patients and are soft, non-tender, and palpated in the cervical, axillary and inguinal regions. Splenomegaly occurs in 10-45% of patients.

Anaemia, leucopenia and thrombocytopenia are common haematological abnormalities seen in SLE. The anaemia may be due to chronic disease, haemolysis (autoimmune or microangiopathic), blood loss, renal insufficiency, drugs, infection, hypersplenism, myelodysplasia, myelofibrosis and aplasia. Autoimmune haemolytic anemia is observed in up to 10% of patients without haemolysis.

Leucopenia (<4500/mm^3) occurs to 30-40% of patients with SLE. Severe leucopenia (neutrophic count <500/mm^3) is rare. Lymphocytopenia (lymphocyte count < 1500/mm^3) is seen in 20% of patients with SLE.

Thrombocytopenia (platelet counts 100 000–150 000/mm^3) is seen in 25-50% of patients and counts of <50 000/mm^3 occur in 10% of patients.

Gastrointestinal (GI) symptoms are seen in 25-40% of patients with SLE. Peritonitis, mesenteric vasculitis with intestinal infarction, pancreatitis and inflammatory bowel disease are rare. Mesenteric thrombosis and infarction may be present in antiphospholipid syndrome. Peptic ulcers are seen in 4-21% of patients, and dyspepsia occurs in 11-50% of patients.

Pancreatitis can be a consequence of vasculitis or thrombosis, and is seen in 2-8% of patients.

Steatosis (excessive fatty infiltration) is secondary to glucocorticoid treatment.

"Lupoid hepatitis" is an autoimmune hepatitis and autoantibodies may help to distinguish this condition from lupus. ANAs are found in both disorders, but anti-smooth muscle and anti-mitochondrial antibodies in SLE are seen in <30% cases only and in low titres. Periportal hepatitis with necrosis is characteristic for autoimmune hepatitis in histopathological examinations.

Ascites is rare in SLE and may be due to congestive heart failure and hypoalbuminaemia secondary to nephritic syndrome or enteropathy causing protein loss.

Ophthalmic symptoms in SLE include retinal vasculitis. It is associated with active systemic disease and presents early in the disease process. Corneal and conjunctiva involvement is part of sicca syndrome and is also associated with SLE. Uveitis, scleritis and optic neuritis are rare manifestations.

THE 1997 REVISED ACR CRITERIA [10]

1. Malar rash – fixed erythema, flat or raised, over the malar eminences, sparing the nasolabial folds.
2. Discoid rash – erythematous raised patches with adherent keratotic scaling and follicular plugging: atrophic scarring may occur in older lesions.
3. Photosensitivity – skin rash as a result of an unusual reaction to sunlight, presented by patient history or observation by physician.
4. Oral ulcers – oral or nasopharyngeal ulceration, usually painless, observed by a physician.
5. Arthritis – nonerosive arthritis involving two or more peripheral joints, characterized by tenderness, swelling or effusion.
6. Serositis:
   a. Pleuritis – convincing history of pleuritic pain or rub heard by a physician or evidence of pleural effusion; or
   b. Pericarditis – documented by ECG or rub or evidence of pericardial effusion.
7. Renal disorder:
   a. Persistent proteinuria greater than 0.5 g per day or greater than 3 + if quantitation not performed.
   b. Cellular casts – may be red cell, hemoglobin, granular, tubular or mixed.
8. Neurologic disorder:
   a. Seizures – in the absence of offending drugs or known metabolic derangement: *e.g.* uremia, ketoacidosis, or electrolyte imbalance
   b. Psychosis – in the absence of offending drugs or known metabolic derangement: *e.g.* uremia, ketoacidosis, or electrolyte imbalance.

  9. Hematologic disorder:
    a. Hemolytic anemia with reticulocytosis; or
    b. Leucopenia – less than 4000/mm^3 or more on two occasions; or
    c. Lymphopenia – less than 1500/mm^3 or more two occasions; or
    d. Thrombocytopenia – less than 100.000/mm^3 in the absence of offending drugs.
 10. Immunologic disorder:
    a. Positive LE cell preparation; or
    b. Anti-DNA: antibody to native DNA in abnormal titers; or
    c. Anti-Sm: presence of antibody to Sm nuclear antigen; or
    d. False positive serologic test for syphilis known to be positive for at least 6 months and confirmed by Treponema pallidum immobilization or fluorescent treponema antibody test.
 11. Antinuclear antibody – an abnormal titer of antinuclear antibodies seen by immunofluorescence or an equivalent assay at any point in time in the absence of offending drugs SLE is confirmed if 4 or more criteria are meet within one is 10 or 11.

2012 SLICC SLE CRITERIA [11]

Clinical Criteria

1. Acute Cutaneous Lupus or Subacute Cutaneous Lupus

Acute cutaneous lupus: lupus malar rash (do not count if malar discoid), bullous lupus, toxic epidermal necrolysis variant of SLE, maculopapular lupus rash, photosensitive lupus rash or

Subacute cutaneous lupus: (nonindurated psoriasiform and/or annular polycyclic lesions that resolve without scarring).

2. Chronic Cutaneous Lupus

Classic discoid rash localized (above the neck) or generalized (above and below the neck), hypertrophic (verrucous) lupus, lupus panniculitis (profundus), mucosal lupus, lupus erythematosus tumidus, chilblains lupus, discoid lupus/lichen planus overlap.

3. Non Scarring Alopecia

Diffuse thinning or hair fragility with visible broken hairs, in the absence of other causes such as alopecia areata, drugs, iron deficiency, and androgenic alopecia.

4. Oral Ulcers or Nasal Ulcers

Oral: palate, buccal, tongue.

Nasal ulcers

In the absence of other causes, such as vasculitis, Behçet's disease, infection (herpesvirus), inflammatory bowel disease, reactive arthritis, and acidic foods.

5. Synovitis

Involving 2 or more joints characterized by swelling or effusion or tenderness in 2 or more joints and at least 30 minutes of morning stiffness.

6. Serositis

Typical pleurisy for more than 1 day OR pleural effusions OR pleural rub.

Typical pericardial pain (pain with recumbency improved by sitting forward) for more than 1 day OR pericardial effusion OR pericardial rub OR pericarditis confirmed by electrocardiography in the absence of other causes, such as infection, uremia, and Dressler's pericarditis.

7. Renal

Urine protein-to-creatinine ratio or (24-hour urine protein) representing $\geq$500 mg protein of more/24 hours OR red blood cell casts.

8. Neurologic

Seizures, psychosis, mononeuritis multiplex (in the absence of other known causes such as primary vasculitis), myelitis, peripheral or cranial neuropathy (in the absence of other known causes such as primary vasculitis, infection, and diabetes mellitus), acute confusional state (in the absence of other causes, including toxic/metabolic, uremia, drugs).

9. Hemolytic Anemia

10. Leukopenia (<4000/mm^3) OR lymphopenia (<1000/mm^3)

Leukopenia at least once: in the absence of other known causes such as Felty's syndrome, drugs, and portal hypertension.

Lymphopenia at least once: in the absence of other known causes such as GCS, drugs, and infection.

11. Thrombocytopenia (<100.000/mm^3)

At least once in the absence of other known causes such as drugs, portal hypertension, and thrombotic thrombocytopenic purpura.

IMMUNOLOGIC CRITERIA

1. **ANA** level above laboratory reference range
2. **Anti-dsDNA** antibody level above laboratory reference range (or 2-fold the reference range if tested by ELISA)
3. **Anti-Sm**: presence of antibody to Sm nuclear antigen
4. **Antiphospholipid antibody** positivity, as determined by
 Positive test for lupus anticoagulant
 False-positive test result for rapid plasma regent
 Medium or high-titer anticardiolipin antibody level (IgA, IgG, or IgM)
 Positive test result for anti-β2 glycoprotein I (IgA, IgG, or IgM).
5. **Low complement** (C3, C4, or CH50)
6. **Direct Coombs'test** (in the absence of hemolytic anemia).

In order to confirm diagnosis of SLE either biopsy-proven lupus nephritis in the presence of ANA OR anti-dsDNA as a "stand-alone" criterion OR four criteria with at least one of the clinical and one of the immunological/ANA criteria.

WHO TYPES OF LUPUS NEPHRITIS [7]

A. Normal glomerulus (class I)
B. Mesangial disease (type II). Mesangial hypercellularity and expansion of the mesangial matrix, which does not compromise capillary loops.
C. Proliferative nephritis. Intense diseases in mesangial and endocapillary cellularity produce a lobular appearance of the glomerular tufts and compromise the patency of capillary loops. When < 50% of glomeruli are involved, it is denoted as focal (type III). When > 50% glomeruli are involved, it is denoted as diffuse (type IV).
D. Membranous nephropathy (type V). Capillary walls of the glomerular tufts are prominent and widely patent resembling "stiff" structures with decreased compliance.

ACTIVITY INDICES

Treatment is defined as disease activity that avoids systemic damage. Several activity indices may be used to evaluate patients with SLE [12], including the European Consensus Lupus Activity Measure [ECLAM], the British Isles Lupus Assessment Group Scale [BILAG], the Lupus Activity Index [LAI], the National Institutes of Health SLE Index Score [SIS], the Systemic Lupus Activity Measure

[SLAM] and the SLE Disease Activity Index [SLEDAI] [SLEDAI-2K or SELENA-SLEDAI versions]. These indices may predict damage and mortality, and reflect changes in disease activity.

The simple index to use is the SLEDAI Index and it includes [13]:

SLEDAI

1. Seizure – 8 points.
2. Psychosis – 8 points.
3. Organic brain syndrome – 8 points.
4. Visual disturbance – 8 points.
5. Cranial nerve disorder – 8 points.
6. Lupus headache – 8 points.
7. CVA (cerebrovascular accident) – 8 points.
8. Vasculitis – 8 points.
9. Arthritis – 4 points.
10. Myositis – 4 points.
11. Urinary casts – 4 points.
12. Haematuria – 4 points.
13. Proteinuria – 4 points.
14. Pyuria – 4 points.
15. Rash – 2 points.
16. Allopecia – 2 points.
17. Mucosal ulcers – 2 points.
18. Pleurisy – 2 points.
19. Pericarditis – 2 points.
20. Low complement – 2 points.
21. Increased DNA binding – 2 points.
22. Fever – 1 points.
23. Thrombocytopenia – 1 points.
24. Leukopenia – 1 points.

Total score 105, severe SLE > 6 points.

CHRONICITY AND DAMAGE INDEX

The SLICC/ACR Damage Index [SDI] is used to evaluate systemic damage caused by SLE [14]. Damage may be due to the disease itself or due to drug treatment, especially glucocorticoids. SDI assess damage in 12 organs or systems. Up to 40-50% of patients with SLE develop damage within 5 years from disease diagnosis, particularly the musculoskeletal system, eyes, skin, cardiovascular, renal and neurological system [14].

DIAGNOSIS

Antinuclear antibodies (ANAs) assay is used to detect connective tissue diseases and has more than 90% sensitivity. Specificity of ANAs for SLE is low, because they are found in other diseases as well as in some healthy people. Autoantibodies to single-stranded DNA (ssDNA) and histones are found in SLE. Antibodies to double-stranded (ds) DNA and anti-Sm (Smith) are specific for SLE patients and found in 70% and 10-30% respectively. Anti-nRNP antibodies are associated with anti-Sm but are not disease specific. Anti-ribosomal antibodies are specific for SLE.

Serum anti-dsDNA titres are associated with LN and progression to end-stage renal disease. Antiphospholipid antibodies are connected with antiphospholipid syndrome. Anti-Ro (SSA) antibodies are associated with neonatal lupus.

MANAGEMENT

Lupus is managed according to disease activity. Improvement in its' treatment is due to improved use of immunosuppressive drugs. Antimalarial drugs are very effective for acute and chronic lupus rashes. Observational studies have suggested that antimalarial drugs such as hydroxychloroquine may be protective against thrombosis. In SLE patients the most common thrombotic events are strokes, followed by deep venous thrombosis. In systemic treatment of mild SLE, such as mild mucocutaneous or musculoskeletal involvement, low-dose glucocorticoids (GCS) (0.1-0.2 mg/kg/day) and antimalarial drugs (HCQ 200 – 400 mg/day) have been used. Prednisone is a predictor of thrombosis.

Most clinical features of SLE may be treated with GCS, however the adverse effects of GCS such as infections, CV diseases and osteoporosis, cause an increase in morbidity. GCS must be tapered and withdrawn and antimalarial drugs must be used instead. Moderate severe SLE (*e.g.* more severe mucocutaneous and musculoskeletal disease or serositis) may be treated with a short-course of medium-dose GCS (0.2-0.5 mg/kg/day), tapered to a lower dose and withdrawn as soon as it is clinically possible.

In patients who are GCS-dependent (*i.e.* whose disease tends to relapse as soon as the dose of GCS is decreased), starting immunosuppressant drug is recommended, *e.g.* for treatment of arthritis, MTX (or LEF); for haematological disease or serositis, AZA or belimumab. Severe lupus *e.g.* proliferative lupus nephritis, CNS involvement or severe thrombocytopenia is treated by pulse IV MP followed by oral GCS (0.5 mg/kg/day) and MMF or IV CYC. Maintenance treatment with a less toxic immunosuppressant agent (AZA, MMF) is used.

GCS improves the prognosis of SLE. Survival rates increased from 50% at 3 years in the mid- XX- century to 92% at 10 years [15]. GCS treatment ranges from low dose (0.1-0.2 mg equivalent prednisolone/kg/day) to moderate (0.2-0.5 mg/kg/day) or high (0.5–1 mg/kg/day) dose, depending on the type of organ involvement.

In the 1970's, intravenous (IV) pulse methylprednisolone (MP) therapy, mostly 500-1000 mg daily for 1-3 days, was introduced [16]. It is very effective in critically ill patients. In the Euro-Lupus Nephritis Trial, after three IV MP daily pulses of 750 mg, patients were switched to oral prednisolone (mostly 0.5 mg/kg/day for 1 month; 1 mg/kg/day in very severe cases), which was tapered by 2.5 mg/day every 2 weeks, to reach a dose of 5 – 7.5 mg/day at 4-6 months [17].

Patients with SLE treated on low-dose GCS for years (2.6-7.5 mg equivalent prednisolone/day) [18] have an increase risk for infection, Cushingoid features, diabetes, cardiovascular effects, myopathy, avascular osteonecrosis, osteoporosis, easy bruising and early cataract. Patients must receive the influenza vaccine (every year) as well as the vaccine for Streptococcal pneumonia (every 5 years) [19].

Antimallarials block toll-like receptor 7 (TLR7) and 9 (TLR9), which are part of the innate immune system. The main antimalarials used to treat lupus are hydroxychloroquine (HQC), chloroquine and quinacrine. Hydroxychloroquine is the drug of choice, it is less likely to cause side effects in the eye, such as retinal damage.

Antimalarials can lower lipid levels, help decrease fatigue, skin rash and diminish joint pain. They act as a blood thinner to decrease the risk of thromboembolic events, have positive effects on patient outcomes and prognosis, spare organs such as the kidneys from damage, prevent thromboembolic disease and decrease the risk of accelerated atherogenesis.

However, lupus patients are only partially responsive to HQC and may need several months of chloroquine, which is five to 10 times stronger than HQC. The use of quinacrine as an alternative to HQC or chloroquine in the management of lupus is not optimal.

Patients with macular degeneration who cannot tolerate chloroquine or HQC may be treated with quinacrine. Quinacrine should be considered in cases of retinal toxicity. Additional benefits may be achieved when combining quinacrine with HQC for patients who do not respond to HQC alone.

HQC leads to reduction in flares, in organ damage, in lipids, in thrombosis, and improvement in survival.

Immunosupresive drugs, especially intravenous cyclophosphamide (CYC), are effective in patients with major organ involvement such as lupus nephritis. Other immunosuppressive drugs used in SLE are azathioprine (AZA) and mycophenolate mofetil (MMF).

The treatment of lupus nephritis (LN) is difficult because only 50% to 70% patients respond well to treatment. The adverse effects of treatment is an additional difficulty [20].

The new guidelines recommend that all patients with clinical evidence of active lupus nephritis should have a renal biopsy performed. Another recommendation is adjunctive treatment that should be given to all patients with lupus nephritis, if possible, including HQC, ACE inhibitors or ARBs [20].

Treatment depends on biopsy results. The guidelines include a treatment algorithm and recommend dosing for improving in various histologic types of lupus nephritis.

Lupus nephritis treatment depends of its severity. Glomerular lesions are graded according to the International Society of Nephrology/Renal Pathology Society (ISN/RPS) classification criteria [7]. Patients with class I or II LN should be treated with angiotensin-converting enzyme inhibitor/angiotensin receptor blockers and HCQ. Patients with proliferative disease (class III and IV) should be treated with immunosuppression.

Three different immunosuppressive regiments can be proposed for patients with class III/IV LN. First NIH IV CYC (0.75-1 g/m^2; every months x 6) combined with IV MP and oral GCS. Second - Euro - Lupus IV CYC (500 mg; every 2 weeks x 6) combined with pulse MP (3 daily pulses of 750 mg) and oral GCS (prednisolone 0.5 mg/kg/day) or third MMF (1-3 g/day ideally 3 g/day. MMF is does not interfere with fertility. Lower response rates to IV CYC (compared with MMF) have been reported in Hispanics and Blacks [20].

Maintenance treatment in LN are AZA (2-2.5 mg/kg/day) and MMF (usually 2 g/day).

Central nervous system involvement must be treated with IV CYC pulse therapy or MMF. CYC is the treatment of choice in patients with organic brain disease, stroke, neuropathies, persistent headache, seizures, psychiatric manifestations, transverse myelitis and cranial neuropathies. Improvement was seen in 61%, stabilization in 29% and deterioration in 10% [21]. CYC was given as monthly pulses (0.75 g/m2) for 6 months and then every 3 months for 1 year.

The only FDA-approved new treatment for lupus is Belimumab. Belimumab is used in seropositive patients with active disease. Belimumab, a fully human monoclonal antibody that inhibits B-lymphocyte stimulator BLYSS, was approved for the treatment of lupus in 2011.

There are many other new therapies in development.

Anti-CD20 rituximab, are used as off-label drugs, with great success in individual patients, but failed in randomized controlled trials [22]. Anti-CD20 orcelizumab or anti-BLYS/APRIL ataçicept, has been associated with a high rate of infections. Epratazumab is an anti CD22 monoclonal antibody that acts as a CD22/B cell receptor (BCR) modulator was first tested in ALLEVIATE-1 and ALLEVIATE-2, which were stopped due to problems with drug supply, but showed some efficacy [23].

Type I interferons (INFs) play an important role in the pathogenesis of SLE. Trials with rontalizumab (anti-INFalpfa), sifalimumab (anti-INFalpha), anti- IL-6 sirukumab, anti IL-6 receptor tocilizumab, abatacept were not found to be better than placebo.

Mortality in SLE is mainly due to infections, complications of atherosclerosis, osteoporosis and malignancies. Haematological malignancies (particularly non-Hodgkin lymphoma), cervical and lung cancer occur more commonly in SLE than in the general population.

NEONATAL LUPUS

Congenital heart block detected before or at birth, in the absence of structural abnormalities, is linked to maternal autoantibodies to Ro(SS-A) and La(SS-B) ribonucleoproteins, regardless of whether the mother has SLE, Sjögren's or is asymptomatic in about 90% of cases. These autoantibodies are also associated with other neonatal abnormalities, such as cutaneous manifestations, cholestasis and cytopenias. Fetal echo Doppler is used to screen pregnancies at risk, usually from 16th to 28th weeks of gestation by determining the PR interval. Treatment of a fetus with complete congenital heart block varies and treatment such as HQC and fetal pacing have all been used, but without definitive proof of efficacy. Complete congenital heart block is not usually reversible and a pacemaker is required. Curative treatment of complete atrioventricular block is based on fluorinated glucocorticoids (betamethason or dexamethasone) that cross the placental barrier, unlike prednisone and methylprednisolone. The value of this treatment is controversial.

ANTIPHOSPHOLIPID SYNDROME (APS)

APS is also known as Hughes' syndrome.

To diagnose of antiphospholipid syndrome (APS), a patient must have both a clinical event (thrombosis or pregnancy loss) and an antiphospholipid antibody (aPL), documented by a solid-phase serum assay (anticardiolipin – aCL), an inhibitor of phospholipid-dependent clotting (lupus anticoagulant – LA), or both.

APS can occur as a single diagnosis, known as primary antiphospholipid antibody syndrome (PAPS), or in association with systemic lupus erythematosus (SLE) or another rheumatic disease and is known as secondary APS (SAPS).

Antiphospholipid antibodies (aPL) can be induced by drugs and by infections. The probability that an asymptomatic person with positive tests for aPL, discovered incidentally, will eventually develop the syndrome is low.

Antiphospholipid antibodies (aPL), (anticardiolipin antibodies (aCL) and lupus anticoagulant (LA) target protein/lipid complexes that are important in the coagulation processes. They predispose to thromboembolic events, thrombocytopenia and pregnancy loss. aPL are antibodies directed at certain serum protein complexes to phospholipid molecules. Abnormally prolonged activated partial thromboplastin time (APTT) is used to screen for aPL. It was originally detected by false-positive tests for syphilis using the Wassermann reaction. Subsequently positive reactivity in the anticardiolipin ELISA assay and in the lupus anticoagulant test was shown to depend on binding of autoantibodies to a serum co-factor, which in the case of the anticardiolipin ELISA is $\beta2$–glycoprotein I ($\beta2$GPI) and in the lupus anticoagulant assay may be either $\beta2$GPI or prothrombin.

Lupus anticoagulants do not function as anticoagulants but as procoagulants by blocking the formation of the prothrombinase complex, resulting in prolonged coagulation assays *in vitro e.g.* prolonged APTT, dilute Russell viper venom time or kaolin clotting time. LA appear not only in SLE but also in primary antiphospholipid syndrome (APS).

Anticardiolipin antibodies (aCL) are detected by ELISA. The most important phospholipid binding protein attaching to the cardiolipin is $\beta2$GPI, which acts as a co-factor in the test. Autoantibodies to $\beta2$GPI and to cardiolipin/$\beta2$GPI complex result positive results which are important to diagnose a procoagulant state. aCL transiently appear in several infections and permanently in syphilis. The antibodies may belong to all three major IgG classes but IgG aCL antibodies are those most closely related to procoagulant activity. Both aCL antibodies and LA can be found in other rheumatic diseases but most commonly in patients with SLE.

Preliminary classification criteria for APS are [24]:

CLINICAL CRITERIA

1. Vascular Thrombosis

One or more episodes of arterial thrombosis or venous thrombosis or small vessel thrombosis, in any tissue or organ confirmed by imaging or Doppler studies or histopathologic studies.

2. Pregnancy Morbidity

  a. One or more unexplained deaths of a morphologically normal fetus at or after the 10th week of gestation with normal fetal morphology or
  b. One or more premature birth of a morphologically normal neonate before the 34th week of gestation because of eclampsia or placental insufficiency or
  c. Three or more unexplained consecutive spontaneous abortion before the 10th week of gestation with anatomic or hormonal abnormalities and paternal and maternal chromosomal causes excluded

LABORATORY CRITERIA

1. Lupus anticoagulant (LA) present in plasma, on two or more occasions at least 12 weeks apart, detected according to the guidelines of the International Society on Thrombosis and Haemostasis (Scientific Subcommittee on LAs/phospholipid – dependent antibodies)
2. Anticardiolipin (aCL) antibody of IgG and/or IgM isotype in serum or plasma, present in medium or high titer (*i.e.* > 40 GPL or MPL, or > the 99th percentile) on two or more occasions, at least 12 weeks apart, measured by a standardized ELISA
3. Anti-beta2-glycoprotein I antibody of IgG and/or IgM isotype in serum or plasma (in titer > the 99 percentile) present on two or more occasions, at least 12 weeks apart, measured by a standardized ELISA, according to recommended procedures.

APS is present if at least one of the clinical criteria and one of the laboratory criteria are met.

Other clinical and laboratory features of the APS are:

Clinical

Livedo reticularis
Thrombocytopenia (usually 50 000 – 100 000 platelets/mm^3)
Autoimmune hemolytic anemia
Cardiac valve disease (vegetations or thickening)
Multiple sclerosis-like syndrome, chorea, or other myelopathy
Laboratory
IgA anticardiolipin antibody
IgA anti-β_2-GPI

Low –titer of antiphospholipid antibody (aPL), usually transient, is found in up to 10% of normal blood donors and moderate-to high-titer anticardiolipin antibody or a positive lupus anticoagulant test in less than 1%.

The prevalence of positive tests increases with age.

PATHOGENESIS

aPL binds mainly to β2GPI. β2GPI is a phospholipids-binding plasma protein present in serum at a concentration of 200 mg/mL and is a member of the complement control protein family with a domain site that activates platelets [25].

Molecular structure of β2GPI domain 5 has a positively charged portion that binds to negatively charged phospholipids of the cellular membrane [25].

β2GPI binds to phosphatidylserine on activated or apoptotic cell membranes of trophoblasts, platelets, and endothelial cells. Under physiological conditions, β2GPI functions in eliminating apoptotic cells and as a natural anticoagulant [25].

Other antigens targeted by aPLs are prothrombin, annexin V, protein C, protein S, kininogens, tissue plasminogen activator, factor VII, factor XI, factor XII and complement component C4. In experimental animal models, immunization with viral and bacterial peptides induces aPLs Ab and clinical events associated with APS [25].

Proposed mechanism of thrombosis and placental injury [25].

Activation or apoptosis of platelets, endothelial cells, or trophoblasts, causes the negatively charged phospholipids phosphatidylserine to migrate from the inner to the outer cell membrane, which is normally electrically neutral. Circulating β2GPI then binds to phosphatydylserine and APL then binds to a β2GPI-phosphatidylserine dimmer [25].

Antiphospholipid antibody – β2GPI dimmer binding activates the extracellular complement cascade; initiates an intracellular, and recruits and activates inflammatory effector cells such as monocytes, neutrophils and platelets, and lead to the release of proinflammatory products (TNF, oxidans, proteases) and the induction of a prothrombotic phenotype. Downregulation of signal transducer and activator of transcription 5 (STAT 5) aPLs inhibit the production of placental prolactin, insulin growth factor binding protein-1, and adversely affect formation of a trophoblast syncytium, placental apoptosis, and trophoblast invasion [25].

Other possible mechanisms of aPL – mediated thrombosis include activation of circulating procoagulant proteins, inhibition of tissue factor expression on monocytes and decrease in fibrinolysis [25].

Deep vein thrombosis and stroke are the most common manifestations of APS.

CLINICAL FEATURES

Clinical features of APS may be asymptomatic but serologically positive (no history of vascular or pregnancy events) to catastrophic APS (multiple thromboses occurring over days).

APS affects all organ systems. Features include recurrent venous or arterial thromboses, pregnancy loss, and catastrophic vascular occlusion. Severity, the young age of affected patients and unusual anatomic locations (Budd-Chiari syndrome and upper extremity thromboses) differ APS thromboses from thromboses caused by other diseases.

Other features include livedo reticularis, thrombocytopenia 50.000 to 100.000 platelets/mm^3, autoimmune hemolytic anemia, cardiac valve disease, multiple sclerosis-like syndrome and other myelopathy, nonfocal neurologic symptoms, chorea, catastrophic vascular occlusion syndrome, pulmonary hypertension, systemic hypertension and renal failure.

OTHER LABORATORY FINDINGS

Immunoglobin A (IgA) anticardiolipin antibody

Antibodies to phosphatidylserine, phosphatidyllinositol, phosphatidyl-glycerol, phosphatidylethanolamine

Proteinuria

False-positive test for syphilis

Hyperintense lesions on T2-weighted brain magnetic resonance imaging.

CATASTROPHIC ANTIPHOSPHOLIPID ANTIBODY SYNDROME

The catastrophic type is the most severe form of APS syndrome.

Features include: clinical evidence of multiple organ involvement that develops over a short period of time (usually less than a week); histopathological features of small vessel occlusions; and laboratory confirmation of the presence of antiphospholipid antibodies.

It is now referred as Asherson's syndrome, described by Ronald Asherson in 1992. Less than 1% of patients with APS develop this variant. The mortality rate is around 30%. Patients with this condition usually end up in intensive care units with multiple organ failure.

PRELIMINARY CRITERIA FOR THE CLASSIFICATION OF CATASTROPHIC APS (CAPS) [26]

1. Evidence of involvement of three or more organs, systems, or tissues.
2. Development of manifestations simultaneously or in less than 1 week.
3. Confirmation by histopathology of small vessel occlusion in at least one organ or tissue.
4. Laboratory confirmation of the presence of antiphospholipid antibody (aPL) (LA or aCL or β2GPI antibodies).
   DEFINITE CATASTROPHIC APS all four criteria.

PROBABLE CATASTROPHIC APS

Criteria 2 through 4 and two organs, systems, or tissues involved.

Criteria 1 through 3, except no confirmation 6 wk apart owing to early death of patient not tested before catastrophic episode.

Criteria 1, 2, and 4.

Criteria 1, 3, and 4 and development of a third event more than 1 week but less than 1 month after the first, despite anticoagulation.

From a histopathological point of view, catastrophic APS is a thrombotic microangiopathic condition.

CATASTROPHIC VASCULAR OCCLUSION

Different diagnosis includes polyarteritis nodosa and disseminated embolization from myxoma, atrial thrombus, or atherosclerotic plaque. Small vessel occlusions occurring in rapid succession suggest disseminated intravascular coagulation. Severe cerebral and renal disease suggest thrombotic thrombocytopenic purpura; renal failure and hemolysis suggest hemolytic-uremic syndrome. APL is rarely present in patients with the alternative diagnosis. Acute adrenal insufficiency is characteristic only in APS and Waterhouse-Friedrichsen syndrome.

Collecting a sufficient amount of patients for epidemiological and clinical research is difficult as CAPS is a rare disease and therefore cooperation between clinical centers is necessary.

The international registry for patients with CAPS

https://ontocrf.costaisa.com/en/web/caps.

Consulting available:

www.med.ub.es/MIMMUN/FORUM/CAPS.HTM

TREATMENT

APS is treated by anticoagulation such as warfarin, heparin, and low-molecula-
-weight heparin, and often in association with low-dose aspirin. Anticoagulation is not indicated for treatment of prophylaxis in asymptomatic seropositive persons. Warfarin is teratogenic therefore only unfractionated or low-molecula-
-weight heparin is used for the treatment of pregnant women. Anticoagulation for thrombosis is started with heparin, followed by long-term maintenance with warfarin, usually at international normalized ratio (INR) of 2.5. Low-dose (81 to 325 mg/day) aspirin, hydroxychloroquine, or both may be added to heparin or warfarin. High doses of GCS are usually given to patients with severe thrombocytopenia, hemolytic anemia, and catastrophic APS syndrome. Subcutaneous heparin, 5000 units twice daily, with low-dose aspirin, increases the fetal survival rate from 50 to 80% in women who have had at least two fetal losses and who test positive for aPL.

Treatment recommendation for APS [27].

Clinical Circumstance	Recommendation
Asymptomatic	No treatment
Venous thrombosis	Warfarin INR 2.5 indifinitely

| Arterial thrombosis | Warfarin INR 2.5 indifinitely |
| Reccurent thrombosis | Warfarin INR 2.5 indifinitely ± low-dose aspirin |

Pregnancy:

First pregnancy	No treatment
Single pregnancy loss at < 10 wk	No treatment
≥1 fetal or ≥3 (pre)-embryonic losses, no thrombosis	Prophylactic heparin + low-dose aspirin throughout pregnancy, discontinue 6-12 wk postpartum
Thromboses regardless of pregnancy history	Therapeutic heparin or low-dose aspirin throughout pregnancy, warfarin postpartum
Valve nodules or deformity	No known effective treatment; full anticoagulation if emboli or intracardiac thrombi demonstrated
Thrombocytopenia > 50 000/mm³	No treatment
Thrombocytopenia < 50 000/mm³	Prednisone, IVIG
Catastrophic antiphospholipid syndrome	Anticoagulation + corticosteroids + IVIG or plasmapheresis

CAPS secondary to SLE is also treated with cyclophosphamide.

Hydroxychloroquine and complement inhibitors have been found to reduce aPL-mediated thrombosis in *in vivo* animal models, while there have been promising human pilot studies showing the benefit of statins and rituximab in treating APS patients [25].

Rivaroxaban a direct factor Xa inhibitor was tested as a treatment of the APS in RAPS trial. Frequent monitoring of its anticoagulant effect is not necessary [25].

Another approach to reduce of aPL activity in APS patients is to inhibit target cell receptors responsible for cell activation such as cell-surface receptor ApoER2', TLR4, Ann A2 and GPIIb/IIIa in aPL-induced activation of Ecs, monocytes and platelets in APS [25].

The preclinical data shows the role of complement activation in the progression of thrombotic and obstetric complications in APS. The inhibition of the complement components C3 and C5 (eculizumab) in *in vivo* murine models have shown to limit the effects of aPL in both thrombotic and obstetric complications [25].

REFERENCES

[1]   Bertsias GK, Pamfil C, Fanouriakis A, Boumpas DT. Diagnostic criteria for systemic lupus erythematosus: has the time come? Nat Rev Rheumatol 2013; 9(11): 687-94.
        [http://dx.doi.org/10.1038/nrrheum.2013.103] [PMID: 23838616]

[2]   Tsokos GC. Systemic lupus erythematosus. N Engl J Med 2011; 365(22): 2110-21.
[http://dx.doi.org/10.1056/NEJMra1100359] [PMID: 22129255]

[3]   Guerra SG, Vyse TJ, Cunninghame Graham DS. The genetics of lupus: a functional perspective.
Arthritis Res Ther 2012; 14(3): 211-34.
[http://dx.doi.org/10.1186/ar3844] [PMID: 22640752]

[4]   Richardson BC, Patel DR. Epigenetics in 2013. DNA methylation and miRNA: key roles in systemic
autoimmunity. Nat Rev Rheumatol 2014; 10(2): 72-4.
[http://dx.doi.org/10.1038/nrrheum.2013.211] [PMID: 24418763]

[5]   Zandman-Goddard G, Solomon M, Rosman Z, Peeva E, Shoenfeld Y. Environment and lupus-related
diseases. Lupus 2012; 21(3): 241-50.
[http://dx.doi.org/10.1177/0961203311426568] [PMID: 22065092]

[6]   Namjou B, Kothari PH, Kelly JA, *et al.* Evaluation of the TREX1 gene in a large multi-ancestral lupus
cohort. Genes Immun 2011; 12(4): 270-9.
[http://dx.doi.org/10.1038/gene.2010.73] [PMID: 21270825]

[7]   Weening JJ, D'Agati VD, Schwartz MM, *et al.* The classification of glomerulonephritis in systemic
lupus erythematosus revisited. Kidney Int 2004; 65(2): 521-30.
[http://dx.doi.org/10.1111/j.1523-1755.2004.00443.x] [PMID: 14717922]

[8]   The American College of Rheumatology nomenclature and case definitions for neuropsychiatric lupus
syndromes. Arthritis Rheum 1999; 42(4): 599-608.
[http://dx.doi.org/10.1002/1529-0131(199904)42:4<599::AID-ANR2>3.0.CO;2-F] [PMID: 10211873]

[9]   Birnbaum J, Petri M, Thompson R, Izbudak I, Kerr D. Distinct subtypes of myelitis in systemic lupus
erythematosus. Arthritis Rheum 2009; 60(11): 3378-87.
[http://dx.doi.org/10.1002/art.24937] [PMID: 19877037]

[10]   Hochberg MC. Updating the American College of Rheumatology revised criteria for the classification
of systemic lupus erythematosus. Arthritis Rheum 1997; 40(9): 1725-33.
[http://dx.doi.org/10.1002/art.1780400928] [PMID: 9324032]

[11]   Petri M, Orbai AM, Alarcón GS, *et al.* Derivation and validation of the Systemic Lupus International
Collaborating Clinics classification criteria for systemic lupus erythematosus. Arthritis Rheum 2012;
64(8): 2677-86.
[http://dx.doi.org/10.1002/art.34473] [PMID: 22553077]

[12]   Urowitz MB, Gladman DD. Measures of disease activity and damage in SLE. Baillieres Clin
Rheumatol 1998; 12(3): 405-13.
[http://dx.doi.org/10.1016/S0950-3579(98)80027-7] [PMID: 9890104]

[13]   Bombardier C, Gladman DD, Urowitz MB, Caron D, Chang CH. Derivation of the SLEDAI. A
disease activity index for lupus patients. Arthritis Rheum 1992; 35(6): 630-40.
[http://dx.doi.org/10.1002/art.1780350606] [PMID: 1599520]

[14]   Gladman DD, Goldsmith CH, Urowitz MB, *et al.* The Systemic Lupus International Collaborating
Clinics/ American College of Rheumatology (SLICC/ARC) damage index for systemic lupus
erythematosus international comparison. J Rheumatol 2000; 27(2): 373-6.
[PMID: 10685799]

[15]   Cervera R, Khamashta MA, Font J, *et al.* Morbidity and mortality in systemic lupus erythematosus
during a 5-year period. A multicenter prospective study of 1,000 patients. Medicine (Baltimore) 1999;
78(3): 167-75.
[http://dx.doi.org/10.1097/00005792-199905000-00003] [PMID: 10352648]

[16]   Cathcart ES, Idelson BA, Scheinberg MA, Couser WG. Beneficial effects of methylprednisolone
"pulse" therapy in diffuse proliferative lupus nephritis. Lancet 1976; 1(7952): 163-6.
[http://dx.doi.org/10.1016/S0140-6736(76)91272-1] [PMID: 54681]

[17]   Houssiau FA, Vasconcelos C, D'Cruz D, *et al.* Immunosuppressive therapy in lupus nephritis: the Euro-Lupus Nephritis Trial, a randomized trial of low-dose versus high-dose intravenous cyclophosphamide. Arthritis Rheum 2002; 46(8): 2121-31.
[http://dx.doi.org/10.1002/art.10461] [PMID: 12209517]

[18]   Buttgereit F, Straub RH, Wehling M, Burmester GR. Glucocorticoids in the treatment of rheumatic diseases: an update on the mechanisms of action. Arthritis Rheum 2004; 50(11): 3408-17.
[http://dx.doi.org/10.1002/art.20583] [PMID: 15529366]

[19]   Naveau C, Houssiau FA. Pneumococcal sepsis in patients with systemic lupus erythematosus. Lupus 2005; 14(11): 903-6.
[http://dx.doi.org/10.1191/0961203305lu2242xx] [PMID: 16335583]

[20]   Houssiau FA, D'Cruz D, Sangle S, *et al.* Azathioprine versus mycophenolate mofetil for long-term immunosuppression in lupus nephritis: results from the MAINTAIN Nephritis Trial. Ann Rheum Dis 2010; 69(12): 2083-9.
[http://dx.doi.org/10.1136/ard.2010.131995] [PMID: 20833738]

[21]   Neuwelt CM, Lacks S, Kaye BR, Ellman JB, Borenstein DG. Role of intravenous cyclophosphamide in the treatment of severe neuropsychiatric systemic lupus erythematosus. Am J Med 1995; 98(1): 32-41.
[http://dx.doi.org/10.1016/S0002-9343(99)80078-3] [PMID: 7825616]

[22]   Merrill JT, Neuwelt CM, Wallace DJ, *et al.* Efficacy and safety of rituximab in moderately-to-severely active systemic lupus erythematosus: the randomized, double-blind, phase II/III systemic lupus erythematosus evaluation of rituximab trial. Arthritis Rheum 2010; 62(1): 222-33.
[http://dx.doi.org/10.1002/art.27233] [PMID: 20039413]

[23]   Wallace DJ, Gordon C, Strand V, *et al.* Efficacy and safety of epratuzumab in patients with moderate/severe flaring systemic lupus erythematosus: results from two randomized, double-blind, placebo-controlled, multicentre studies (ALLEVIATE) and follow-up. Rheumatology (Oxford) 2013; 52(7): 1313-22.
[http://dx.doi.org/10.1093/rheumatology/ket129] [PMID: 23542611]

[24]   Miyakis S, Lockshin MD, Atsumi T, *et al.* International consensus statement on an update of the classification criteria for definite antiphospholipid syndrome (APS). J Thromb Haemost 2006; 4(2): 295-306.
[http://dx.doi.org/10.1111/j.1538-7836.2006.01753.x] [PMID: 16420554]

[25]   Willis R, Harris EN, Perangeli S. The future of treatment for antiphospholipid syndrome. Int J Clin Rheumatol 2014; 9: 41-57.
[http://dx.doi.org/10.2217/ijr.13.73]

[26]   Asherson RA, Cervera R, de Groot PG, *et al.* Catastrophic antiphospholipid syndrome: international consensus statement on classification criteria and treatment guidelines. Lupus 2003; 12(7): 530-4.
[http://dx.doi.org/10.1191/0961203303lu394oa] [PMID: 12892393]

[27]   Espinosa G, Cervera R. Thromboprophylaxis and obstetric management of the antiphospholipid syndrome. Expert Opin Pharmacother 2009; 10(4): 601-14.
[http://dx.doi.org/10.1517/14656560902772302] [PMID: 19284363]

CHAPTER 5

Sjögren's or Sicca Syndrome and Mikulicz's Disease or an IgG4-Related Disease

Abstract: Sjögren's or sicca syndrome (SS), is a progressive, inflammatory autoimmune disease affecting the exocrine glands. Clinical features include mucosal dryness presented as xerophthalmia (keratoconjuctivitis sicca), xerostomia, xerotrachea and vaginal dryness, major salivary gland enlargement, non-erosive polyarthritis and Raynaud's phenomenon. The symptoms are mild from dryness of mucosal surfaces in some patients to very severe with involvement of many organs in others. The disease has increased mortality, due to extraglandular systemic involvement and often accompanying lymphoma. Laboratory tests show positive antinuclear antibodies, rheumatoid factor and anti Ro/SSA, anti La/SSB antibodies. Biopsy of the minor salivary glands is a gold standard in the diagnosis of SS. The focus score in an area of 4 mm^2 describes focal aggregates of at least 50 lymphocytes. One present focus score represents a positive result. Structural damage on the eye surface is evaluated using the Lissamine green test.

Patients with SS have a 44 times higher risk of developing lymphoma than normal control population.

Extraglandular symptoms may be treated with GCS and immunosuppresive drugs in severe cases (CYC, AZA or MMF in pulmonary alveolitis, glomerulonephritis or severe neurological features).

Mikulicz's disease (MD) is an IgG4-related disease. Criteria of MD are: increased IgG4 level (>135 mg/dl), tissue biopsy with infiltration of IgG4 plasmocytes with fibrosis and sclerosis.

Differences between MD and SS: MD does not show the same female predominance. Allergic rhinitis and autoimmune pancreatitis are seen more often in MD. There is an increased improvement after GCS treatment in patients with MD than with SS.

Keywords: Anti La/SSB antibodies, Anti Ro/SSA antibodies, Exocrine glands, Focus score, IgG4 level, IgG4-related disease, Keratoconjuctivitis sicca, Lymphoma, Major salivary gland enlargement, Mikulicz's disease, Mucosal dryness, Non-erosive polyarthritis, Raynaud's phenomenon, Sicca syndrome, Sjögren's syndrome, Xerophthalmia, Xerostomia, Xerotrachea.

INTRODUCTION

Sjögren's known as Sicca Syndrome (SS), is a slowly progressive, inflammatory autoimmune disease affecting the exocrine glands. Lymphocytes replace functional epithelium in exocrine glands, causing decreased secretions (exocrinopathy) such as oral dryness (xerotomia), eye dryness (xerophthalmia), dryness of the nose, pharynx and vagina. Characteristic autoantibodies, anti-Ro (SS-A) and anti-La (SS-B) are produced. The symptoms are mild from dryness of mucosal surfaces in some patients to very severe with involvement of many organs in others. Different symptoms of SS in individuals delay diagnosis up to 10 years. This disease has increased mortality, due to extraglandular systemic involvement and often accompanying lymphoma.

PSS occurs secondly to rheumatoid arthritis and other diseases. The diagnosis of SS is difficult and require a multidisciplinary consultation. Sicca symptoms are common, non-specific, and there is no gold standard diagnostic test.

Professor Henrik Sjögren was an ophtalmonologist, who first described the association of dry mouth, keratoconjuctivitis sicca, and rheumatoid arthritis in 1933 and this syndrome was named after him.

EPIDEMIOLOGY

Primary Sjögren's syndrome is the most common autoimmune diseases, with a prevalence ranging from 0.1 to 4.6%, female: male = 9: 1. Onset usually occurs in the 4th -5th decade of life. PSS affects predominantly middle-aged women [1]. It occurs in 4% of population. In male patients with sicca symptoms it is very important to exclude IgG4 related disease.

Sicca Manifestations of Sjögren's Syndrome

Clinical features of SS include mucosal dryness presented xerophthalmia (keratoconjuctivitis sicca), xerostomia, xerotrachea and vaginal dryness.

Non-sicca Manifestations of Sjögren's Syndrome

Clinical features include chronic fatigue, fever of unknown origin, leucocytoclastic vasculitis, major salivary gland enlargement due to parotid or submandibular gland swelling, Raynaud's phenomenon without teleangiectasia or digital ulcerations, non-erosive polyarthritis, peripheral neuropathy, renal tubular acidosis of unknown origin, pulmonary fibrosis.

The periepithelial extraglandular manifestations due to the infiltration of lymphocytes into epithelial tissues of lungs, kidneys and liver; they appear early in the disease and have a benign course. The extraepithelial manifestations, such as skin vasculitis, peripheral neuropathy and glomerulonephritis, with low C4 levels, are associated with an increased morbidity and a high risk for lymphoma.

Laboratory tests show raised erythrocyte sedimentation rate, hypergamma-globulinaemia, leucopenia and thrombocytopenia, positive antinuclear antibodies, rheumatoid factor and anti Ro/SSA, anti La/SSB antibodies.

Primary Sjögren's Syndrome (PSS) has more criteria than any other rheumatic condition. 12 sets of classification criteria have been proposed since the mid-1980s.

CLASSIFICATION CRITERIA FOR SS: Copenhagen 1986, Greek 1986, Californian (San Diego) 1986, Japanese I 1986, European I 1993, European II 1996, Japanese II 1997, Japanese III 2000, American-European 2002, SICCA-ACR 2012, ACR/EULAR criteria 2016.

In 2012 Shiboski *et al.* [2], proposed a new set of classification criteria for SS on behalf of the American College of Rheumatology (ACR) criteria. These differ from the AECG criteria from 2002 in the exclusion of some sicca symptoms and diagnostic tests of salivary glands and the modification of others like inclusion of a new ocular staining score and ANA and RF in the immunological criteria.

SICCA-ACR 2012 classification criteria have been published based on data from the International Collaborative Clinical Alliance Cohort. These criteria are from objective test results and at least 2 of the following are required to classify PSS:

1. Positive serum anti-Ro/SS-A and/or anti-La/SS-B antibodies or (positive rheumatoid factor and antinuclear antibody titer $\geq$1: 320);
2. Labial salivary gland biopsy exhibiting focal lymphocytic sialadenitis with a focus score $\geq$1 focus/4 mm^2.
3. Keratoconjuctivitis sicca with ocular staining score $\geq$3 (assuming that the individual is not currently using daily eye drops for glaucoma and has not had corneal surgery or cosmetic eyelid surgery in the last 5 years).

2016 ACR/EULAR Classification Criteria for Primary Sjögren's Syndrome are [3]:

Labial salivary gland with focal lymphocytic sialadenitis and focal score of $\geq$ 1 foci/4 mm^2	3
Anti-SS-A/Ro positive	3
Ocular Staining Score (OSS) $\geq$ 5 (or van Bijsterveld score $\geq$ 4) in at least 1 eye	1
Schirmer's test $\leq$ 5 mm/5 minutes in at least 1 eye	1

Unstimulated whole saliva flow rate (UWS) ≤ 0.1 ml/min   1

Total score ≥ 4 diagnose is confirmed if any individual who meets the inclusion criteria and does not have any of the conditions listed as exclusion criteria.

The inclusion criteria can be applied to any patient with at least 1 symptom of ocular or oral dryness as a positive response to at least 1 of the following questions:

1. Have you had daily persistent, troublesome dry eyes for more than 3 months?
2. Do you have a recurrent sensation of sand or gravel in the eyes?
3. Do you use tear substitutes more than 3 times a day?
4. Have you had a daily feeling of dry mouth for more than 3 months?
5. Do you frequently drink liquids to aid in swallowing dry food?

The exclusion criteria include prior diagnosis of any of the following conditions?

1. History of head and neck radiation treatment
2. Active hepatitis C infection
3. AIDS
4. Sarcoidosis
5. Amyloidosis
6. Graft versus host disease
7. IgG4-related disease

Genetic Predisposition: Antigen HLA DR3, HLA DR4, HLA DRw52, and HLA B8.

ETIOLOGY of SS are bacteria, viruses (Epstein Barr virus, cytomegalovirus, hepatitis C virus, retroviruses), hormonal disorders.

Pathogenesis

In the pathogenesis of SS, genetic and environmental factors play a role. In B cell differentiation and activation, polymorphism of the early B cell factor 1, B cell lymphocyte kinase and tumor necrosis factor superfamily member 4 (TNFSF4) genes are associated with disease susceptibility [4]. With primary SS, gene polymorphism of interferon regulatory factor-5 and a transcription factor involved in IFN signaling pathway is associated [5]. Other important mediators of type I INF action are alleles of IFN regulatory factor-5 and STAT-4 [6]. Activation of the pathways of INFs, by antiviral proteins against viruses (Epstein-Barr virus, herpesviruses, coxsackie virus, retroviruses and hepatitis C virus) describe the viral hypothesis. The prevalence of women in their postmenopause years suggests that hormonal factors may influence disease activation.

In the pathogenesis of SS epithelial cells are important. They produce varied cytokines, chemokines, and molecules which are able to start local immune responses (HLA class II, costimulatory molecules) [7].

Lymphocytes also play an important role in the pathogenesis of primary SS. The main cells that invade are CD4+ T lymphocytes [8]. B cells in the lesions contain intracytoplasmic immunoglobulins with anti-Ro (SSA) and/or anti-La (SSB) reactivity [9]. The predisposing factor for oligoclonal B lymphocytes and lymphoma are germinal centre formation in salivary infiltrates [10].

Macrophages and plasmacytoid dendritic cells with Toll-like receptors 7 and 9 produce INF suggesting that the presence of a viral or viral-like trigger at salivary gland tissue. INFs express B cell activating factor of the TNF family (BAFF) or B lymphocyte stimulator (BLyS) by monocytes, dendritic cells and salivary gland epithelial cells [11]. T and B cell-attracting chemokines together with BAFF produce a micro-environment that enhance B cell aggregation and differentiation, and local production of anti-SSA/SSB antibodies [12]. B cells produce immunoglobulins and autoantibodies. Stimulation of B cells may lead to the development of lymphoma in patients with primary SS.

Chronic infection of the epithelial cells by a virus increase INF production [13] which may result in further activation of epithelial salivary cells leading to exposure of antigens such as Ro/SSA and La/SSB and production of anti Ro/SSA and anti La/SSB antibodies [14].

Hyperactivity of B lymphocytes and lymphocytic infiltration of the lacrimal glands and salivary glands are observed.

Plasmacytoid dendritic cells and regulatory B cells are aberrant and leads to disregulation of T cells and B cells, the loss of immunologic tolerance to self-antigens, and abnormal regulation of oestrogens and androgens.

Glandular hypofunction results from downregulation of receptor-mediated secretion of salivary fluid into the ductal lumen. Glandular hypofunction might include: blockade of M3R by autoantibodies, inhibition of intracellular signaling pathway involved in the fluid secretory process, altered expression of aquaporin 5 (AQP5), which is responsible for water movement. The periepithelial extraglandular manifestations are the results of lymphocytic invasion in epithelial tissues of the lung, kidneys and liver. They appear early in the disease and have a benign course.

Examinations of the Mouth

The gold standard in diagnosing is biopsy of the minor salivary glands using the lower lip [15]. The focal score in an area of 4 mm^2 is investigated under microscopic examinations. It describes focal aggregates of at least 50 lymphocytes and one present focus score results in a positive result according to the Greenspain's scale [16]. A recent consensus published guidelines as to how to obtain the samples and the types of samples to be sent for histopathological analysis [17].

General Guidance

1. The minimum number of minor salivary glands is suggested to be four (six if small), and should be surgically separated.
2. The minimum surface area of gland sections examined should be 8 mm^2.
3. If the first cutting level is inconclusive, or in the context of a clinical trial, two additional cutting levels at 200 um intervals (typical focus diameter is <50um) in order to increase the surface area should be considered.
4. Paraffin blocks should be prepared with care, and smaller glands set higher to allow mid-specimen sampling during cutting.
5. Histological examination should determine whether there is FLS present. Attribution of FLS (focal lymphocytic sialadenitis), or possible FLS, should be followed by calculation of a focus score.
6. The extent (absent, mild, moderate, severe) of atrophy, fibrosis, duct dilatation and non-specific chronic sialadenitis, in addition to the presence or absence of FLS, should be reported.
7. Calculation of the focus score should include the whole of the glandular surface area in the denominator, to avoid introduction of bias.
8. The presence or absence of germinal centre-like structures and lymphoepithelial lesions should be reported [17].

A protocol for analysis of minor salivary gland biopsies is available on the Sjogren's International Collaborative Clinical Alliance consortium website: http://sicca.ucsf.edu/Labial_Salivary_Gland_Assessment.doc

Unstimulated sialometry <=1.5 mL/15 min, or 0.1 mL/min is decreased. Stimulated sialometry may be tested 5 min after the unstimulated sialometry, using paraffin chewing gums or lemon juice. Patients should deposit saliva into a test tube every minute for 15 minutes, accumulating of saliva < 1.5 mL [18].

Parotid scintigraphy [19] grades the involvement of major salivary glands into four categories, with IV representing severe involvement at diagnosis, and is associated with a higher risk of lymphoma and death [20].

Ultrasonography is a non-invasive test used to assess parotid enlargement [21].

Examinations of the Eyes

Schirmer's tear test- a strip of filter paper 30 mm in length is slipped under the lower lid. After 5 minutes the wetting length of the paper is measured. Wetting less than 5 mm over 5 minutes is a strong indication of diminished secretion.

Rose Bengal staining – the cornea is examined by a slit-lamp, and shows a punctuate or filamentary keratitis.

Structural damage of the eye surface is evaluated using the Lissamine green test which replaced the painful Rose Bengal test. If the epithelium is damaged the cornea and conjunctiva are stained green. Each area of the eye (nasal, central, temporal) is scored from 0 to 3. The sum of the different scores from 0 to 9 for each eye represents the van Bijsterveld score. The score is ≥4 in both eyes is diagnostic.

Clinical Feature of Sjögren's Syndrome

Glandular Involvement

Mouth dryness is due to decreased salivary secretion because of involvement of the major and minor salivary glands. This may cause oral infections, mucosal damage and dental caries due to loss of the lubricating, buffering and antimicrobial qualities of saliva. Fungal infections, especially candidiasis, are also common.Fissured tongue and atrophy of filiform papillae are seen. Oral dryness occurs in >95% of patients.

Sensation of ocular dryness gives the feeling of itching, grittiness, soreness and dryness, photosensitivity, erythema, eye fatigue or decreased visual acuity. Decreased tear secretion leads to chronic irritation and destruction of corneal and bulbar conjunctival epithelium (keratoconjuctivitis sicca). Ocular infections, such as blepharitis, bacterial keratitis, conjunctivitis and corneal ulcerations may be observed.

Decreased saliva volume cause dysphagia. Reduction of respiratory tract glandular secretions cause dryness of the nose, throat and trachea, and a non-productive cough [22]. Involvement of the exocrine glands of the skin leads to cutaneous dryness. In female patients with SS, dryness of the vagina and vulva may result in dyspareunia and pruritis, affecting quality of life.

Fatigue, generalized pain, weakness, sleep disturbances, anxiety and depression are very common [23]. Polyarthralgia and myalgia are seen in more than 50% of patients.

Symmetrical joint involvement of hands and arthritis was observed in 53% of patients [24]. The arthritis of PSS is non-erosive, joint deformity is rare and myalgias are often seen.

Skin dryness is common, and in 10% of patients small-vessel vasculitis is observed [22] represented as cutaneous purpura. Sometimes nodules, digital lesions or maculopapular rash and cutaneous ulcers are observed. Cryoglobulins were positive in one-third of cases and vasculitis was confirmed by biopsy in nearly half; 90% has leucocytoclastic vasculitis. Annular erythema occurred less frequently [25].

Raynaud's phenomenon in pSS is milder than in other systemic autoimmune disease such as SSc with digital loss, digital pulp pitting or fingertip infarctions. Cardiac involvement is rare.

Pulmonary arterial hypertension in PSS is observed in 22% [26].

Gastrointestinal involvement includes oesophageal motility, chronic gastritis and malabsorption. 20-30% of patients have abnormal liver function tests. Renal involvement is rare. Tubulointerstitial nephritis, which is caused by type I renal tubular acidosis is an early manifestations of SS. The main features of renal tubular acidosis is hypokalaemia and renal colic due to nephrocalcinosis. Diabetes insipidus and renal failure may also be observed, as well as glomerulonephritis with nephritic syndrome. Patients with glomerulonephritis present with cryoglobulins, usually type II – mixed monoclonal, containing an IgMk monoclonal rheumatoid factor. Renal biopsy shows membranoproliferative, mesangioproliferative or membranous glomerulonephritis.

Cystitis with urinary tract infection with poliuria and nycturia is observed [27].

Peripheral neuropathy has been reported in 10% of PSS [28]. They are sensory and sensorimotor axonal polyneuropathy related to lowest frequency of immunological markers of SS but multiplex mononeuropathy is associated with a high disease activity. The most disabling is pure sensory neuropathy, which a characteristic neurological complication of PSS, caused by damage of the sensory neurons of the dorsal root and gasserian ganglia.

Patients with SS may have cranial nerve involvement (the trigeminal (V), vestibulocochlear (VIII) and facial (VII) cranial pairs). Trigeminal neuralgia is a common complication of PSS seen in about 15% of patients [29].

Severe central nervous system involvement in patient with PSS is rare. Some patients may develop aseptic meningitis of myelitis with or without optic neuritis [30].

Lymphoproliferative Disease

Patients with primary sicca syndrome have a 44 times higher relative risk of developing lymphoma than the age-, sex- and race-matched normal control population. The majority of lymphomas are extranodal marginal zone B cell lymphomas of mucosa. In most cases, lymphoid tissue (MALT) type is associated.

Lymphomas that develop in patients with PSS are extranodal in 80% of cases, mostly in the parotid glands [31]. Persistently hard enlargement of the parotid gland or less frequently of the lacrimal glands, should raise suspition of lymphoma. Lymphomas developing in SS may also occur in the gastrointestinal tract or lungs. Mucosa-associated lymphoid tissue lymphomas are the most common type, followed by marginal zone lymphomas.

Risk factors for lymphoma include severe parotid involvement, purpura, cryoglobulins, monoclonal band and hypocomplementaemia [32].

Laboratory Examination

Rising ESR over 100, anemia, leucopenia with lymphopenia, thrombocytopenia, hypergammaglobulinemia, RF positive, antinuclear antibodies, anti-Ro (SS-A), anti-La (SS-B), cryoglobulinemia, immunological complexes, antimitochondrial antibodies, anti-tyreoglobulin antibodies, antibodies – anti-epithelium and salivary duct, antibodies – anti-DNA, anti-Sm, anti-histons, anti-RNP – in secondary sicca syndrome are observed.

C-reactive protein levels are usually normal [22].

One of the most characteristic laboratory abnormalities in PSS is polyclonal hypergammaglobulinemia. It represents the polyclonal B cell activation. Hypergammaglobulinemia is closely associated with immunological markers of SS (RF, anti Ro/SSA and anti-La/SSB) [32].

ANA (antinuclear antibodies) are the most frequently detected antibodies in PSS (in >80% of cases) [33].

Ani-Ro/SSA and La/SSB antibodies are detected in 30-70% of patients and are associated with extraglandular features [34]. Sometimes negative anti Ro/SSA antibodies accompany positive anti-Ro52 antibodies [33].

In about 10% of cases, PSS may present with circulating mixed cryoglobulins [32]. Patients with cryoglobulinaemia are at a higher risk of B cell lymphoma [35].

In patients with PSS hypocomplementaemia is found in 10-25% of patients [32].

Primary and Secondary Sicca Syndrome

Clinical features of primary and secondary sicca syndrome are the same. Primary Sjögren's is diagnosed after the exclusion of other rheumatic diseases. Secondary Sjögren's is diagnosed when there is accompanying evidence of another connective tissue disease, most frequently rheumatoid arthritis or others like systemic lupus erythematosus, systemic sclerosis, polymyositis) and with autoimmunologic diseases (primary biliary cirrhosis, autoimmune hepatitis, autoimmune thyroiditis) were observed.

Other causes of enlargement of salivary glands are: acute viral infection, acute bacterial infection, tuberculosis, actinomycosis, benign or malignant primary gland tumor, Waldenstrom' macroglobulinemia, sarcoidosis, hyperlipidemia IV and V, cirrhosis hepatitis, diabetes mellitus, and hypersensitivity to iodine, lead or copper.

Suspicion of lymphoma: enlargement of ganglia, splenomegaly, hepatomegaly, enlargement of salivary glands, vasculitis, fever, weight loss, purpura, low C4, cryoglobulinemia.

Validated Outcome Measures

The EULAR Sjögren's Syndrome Patients Reported Index (ESSPRI) is a patient questionnaire to assess subjective symptoms.

The EULAR Sjögren's Syndrome Disease Activity Index (ESSDAI) it is a systemic activity index to assess systemic complications [36].

EULAR Sjögren's Syndrome Disease Activity Index (ESSDAI) [36]

The EULAR Sjögren's Syndrome Disease activity Index (ESSDAI) domain.

DOMAIN

Constitutional (exclusion of fever of infectious origin and voluntary)

Weight loss

Lymphadenopathy (exclusion of infection)

Glandular (exclusion of stone or infection)

Articular (exclusion of osteoarthritis)

Cutaneous

Pulmonary

Renal

PNS

CNS

Haematological

Biological

The European League Against Rheumatism (EULAR) Sjögren's Syndrome Patients Reported Index (ESSPRI) [37]. The total score is the mean score of the 3 scales.

1. How severe has your dryness been during the last 2 weeks?
2. How severe has your fatigue been during the last 2 weeks?
3. How severe has your pain (joint or muscular pains in your arms or legs) been during the last 2 weeks?

DIFFERENTIAL DIAGNOSIS

The most common cause of sicca features is treatment with antihypertensive, antihistamine and antidepressant drugs.

Other causes include allergy/atopy, infections, dehydration or irradiation. Chronic viral infections (HCV or HIV)

Systemic diseases (sarcoidosis and tuberculosis), amyloid proteins (amyloids) or malignant cells (haematological neoplasia) and IgG4-RD.

MANAGEMENT OF SJÖGREN'S SYNDROME

Local Treatment of Dry Eyes

1. Patient education.
2. Use of moisturizing drops (such as glucan containing sodium hyaluronate and hydroxypropylmethylcellulose).
3. Use of artificial tears.
4. Closed lacrimal points.
5. Avoid GCS drops.
6. Use of ciclosporin drops (0.05% CsA drops twice daily).

Local Treatment of Dry Mouth

1. Intensive oral hygiene.
2. Stimulation of basal saliva secretion.
3. Fluorine supplementation.
4. Use special tooth paste.
5. Use artificial saliva.
6. Drinking sips of water instead of big quantities, reduces dry mouth symptoms without nocturia.

The use of anticholinergic drugs, alcohol and smoking is contradictory while water intake, mechanical stimulation with sugar-free gums and candies, and fluoride toothpaste may improved the quality of life.

Systemic Treatment

There is currently a lack of disease-modifying drugs in PSS. Fatigue, myalgia, and arthralgia/arthritis do not respond to hydroxychloroquine.

Extraglandular symptoms may be treated with GCS and immunosuppresive drugs in severe cases.

Cyclophosphamide(CYC), azathioprine (AZA) or mycophenolate mofetil (MMF) may be used in pulmonary alveolitis, glomerulonephritis or severe neurological features.

Pulmonary hypertension may be treated with an endothelin receptor antagonist, inhibitor of type 5 phosphodiesterase and prostanoids.

Renal tubular acidosis – K supplementation, sodium bicarbonate against acidosis, which prevents formation of stones in the kidney.

Diabetes insipidus – diuretics, low sodium and low protein diet.

Peripheral neuropathy –GCS. Cranial neuropathy – GCS and gabapentin or carbamazepine, duloxetine. CNS involvement – GCS in pulses + immunosuppression. Gamma globulins or rituximab.

Esophageal dysmotility – metoclopramide, domperidon, erythromycin. GERD (gastroesophageal reflux disease) – proton pump inhibitor (PPI).

Primary biliary cirrhosis – ursodeoxycholic acid, hydroxychloroquine.

Rash – GCS, hydroxychloroquine, dapsone, methotrexate, azathioprine. Purpura – GCS, immunosuppressive treatment, sometimes plasmapheresis.

Two oral secretors stimulate saliva and tear flow. They are muscarinic agonists (pilocarpine and cevimeline) and stimulate the M1 and M3 receptors present on salivary glands, leading to increased secretory function.

Pilocarpine (Salogen) stimulates the M3R, and is given in a 5 mg dose three to four times daily and improves measures of both dry eyes and dry mouth. Cevimeline (Evoxac) also stimulates the M3R and improves measures of dry eyes and mouth. Cevimeline must be used in doses of 30 mg per 8 hours. Pilocarpine and cevimeline are contraindicated in patients with iritis, narrow angle glaucoma, and moderate – to-severe asthma. In patients with intolerance to muscarinic agonists, N-acetylcysteine may be used instead.

Biologic Treatment

More than 20 studies have analysed the use of seven biological agents in PSS: IFN alpha, two anti-TNF agents (infliximab – a monoclonal antibody against TNF, and etanercept – a recombinant soluble TNF receptor), three B cell targeted therapies (rituximab – a monoclonal antibody against CD20, epratuzumab – a monoclonal antibody against CD22, and belimumab – a monoclonal antibody against BAFF) and a T cell targeted therapy (abatacept). Randomised controlled trials have shown the lack of efficacy of anti-TNF agents and controversial results for B-cell-depleting agents [38].

Methylprednisolone and CYC pulses should be used in patients with severe systemic vasculitis or CNS involvement, with plasma exchange being added in severe cases [20].

MIKULICZ's Disease (MD) is an IgG4-related syndrome or IgG4 positive multiple organ lymphoproliferative syndrome (IgG4+MOLPS). Originally it was considered part of Sjögren's syndrome, but recently it has been reclassified as an

IgG4-positive multiple organ lymphoproliferative syndrome (IgG4+MOLPS) [39].

Diagnostic criteria of Mikulicz's disease are:

Decreased level of IgG4 (>135 mg/dl)

Tissue biopsies with infiltration of IgG4 plasmocytes (>50%) with fibrosis and sclerosis, and rarely lymphocytic infiltration in epithelial gland ducts [39].

In 1888 Jan Mikulicz-Radecki described a man with symmetric lacrimal, submandibular and parotid gland edema of unknown etiology. In a histopathological exam of the edematous lacrimal gland he discovered massive mononuclear cell infiltration. The disease was later named after him.

In 1953 Morgan *et al.* described that Mikulicz disease was not a distinct disease but only a manifestation of SS. However, between 1960 and 2006 more than 20 cases of MD were described in Japan, and some differences between MD and SS have been reported [39].

Differences between Mikulicz's disease and Sjögren's syndrome:

1. IgG4-related syndromes have do not show the same female predominance.
2. Patients with Mikulicz's disease have significantly more enlarged lacrimal and salivary glands but a lower frequency of dry eyes and mouth.
3. More complications such as autoimmune pancreatitis are described in Mikulicz's disease.
4. Allergic rhinitis is seen significantly more often in Mikulicz's disease as well as autoimmune pancreatitis, and serum levels of IgG1, IgG2, IgG4 and IgE level all of which are significantly higher in comparison with SS patients.
5. There is an increased clinical improvement after GCS treatment in patients with Mikulicz's disease than in patients with Sjögren's syndrome.

IgG4 related diseases are:

- Type 1 autoimmune pancreatitis or AIP (IgG4-related pancreatitis).
- IgG4-related sclerosing cholangitis.
- Mikulicz's disease (IgG4-related dacryoadenitis and sialadenitis).
- Sclerosing sialadenitis (Kuttner's tumor, IgG4-related submandibular gland disease).
- Inflammatory orbital pseudotumor (IgG4-related orbital inflammation or orbital inflammatory pseudotumor).
- Chronic sclerosing dacryoadenitis (lacrimal gland enlargement, IgG4-related dacryoadenitis).

- A subset of patient with "idiopathic" retroperitoneal fibrosis (Ormond's disease) and related disorers (IgG4-related retroperitoneal fibrosis, IgG4-related mesenteritis).
- Chronic sclerosing aortitis and periaortitis (IgG4-related aortitis or periaortitis).
- Riedelo's thyroiditis (IgG4-related thyroid disease).
- IgG4-related interstitial pneumonitis and pulmonary inflammatory pseudotumors (IgG4-related lung disease).
- IgG4-related kidney disease (including tubulointerstitial nephritis and membranous glomerulonephritis secondary to IgG4-related diseases).
- IgG4-related hypophysitis.
- IgG4-related pachymeningitis.

The incidence of xerostomia, xerophthalmia and arthralgia, rheumatoid factor an antinuclear, antySS-A/Ro and anti SSB/La antibodies was significantly lower in patients with MD than in those with typical SS. Histological samples from patients with MD showed marked IgG4 plasma cell infiltration. Many patients with MD had lymphocytic follicle formation, but lymphoepithelial lesions were rare.

In women with MD IgG4, IgG, IgG2 and IgE were significantly higher than in typical SS. In contrast IgG1, IgG3, IgA and IgM levels were significantly lower in MD than in typical SS.

Patients with MD showed lymphocyte and IgG4 plasma cell infiltration with fibrosis (sclerotic lesions).

Tissue biopsies showed infiltration of IgG4 plasmocytes (>50%) with fibrosis and sclerosis, but rarely lymphocytic infiltration in epithelial gland ducts [38]. Lymphocytic follicle formation was also observed. Lymphocytic infiltration into the ducts (formation of lymphoepithelial lesions) was rare in comparison to SS [39].

Swollen glands are usually correlated with xerostomia and xerophthalmia in patients with SS. Xerostomia and xerophthalmia was significantly lower in patients with MD than in SS, even in cases where the lacrimal, parotid or submandibular glands were swollen. Histopathological examination showed that lymphocytic infiltration in the ducts and formation of lymphoepithelial lesions are rare in MD, even in cases with severe lymphocyte and plasma cell expansion. This explains the swelling of the glands without dryness in MD [39].

REFERENCES

[1]   Qin B, Wang J, Yang Z, *et al.* Epidemiology of primary Sjögren's syndrome: a systematic review and meta-analysis. Ann Rheum Dis 2015; 74(11): 1983-9.

[http://dx.doi.org/10.1136/annrheumdis-2014-205375] [PMID: 24938285]

[2]   Shilboski SC, Shiboski CH, Criswell LA, *et al.* American College of Rheumatology Classification Criteria for Sjögren's syndrome: a data-driven, expert consensus approach in the SICCA cohort. Arthritis Care Res (Hoboken) 2012; 64: 475-87.
[http://dx.doi.org/10.1002/acr.21591] [PMID: 22563590]

[3]   Shiboski CH, Shiboski SC, Seror RS, *et al.* American College of Rheumatology/ European League Against Rheumatism Classification Criteria for Primary Sjögren's Syndrome. Arthritis Rheum 2016; 2016
[http://dx.doi.org/10.1002/art.39859]

[4]   Nordmark G, Kristjansdottir G, Theander E, *et al.* Association of EBF1, FAM167A(C8orf13)-BLK and TNFSF4 gene variants with primary Sjögren's syndrome. Genes Immun 2011; 12(2): 100-9.
[http://dx.doi.org/10.1038/gene.2010.44] [PMID: 20861858]

[5]   Miceli-Richard C, Comets E, Loiseau P, Puechal X, Hachulla E, Mariette X. Association of an IRF5 gene functional polymorphism with Sjögren's syndrome. Arthritis Rheum 2007; 56(12): 3989-94.
[http://dx.doi.org/10.1002/art.23142] [PMID: 18050197]

[6]   Nordmark G, Kristjansdottir G, Theander E, *et al.* Additive effects of the major risk alleles of IRF5 and STAT4 in primary Sjögren's syndrome. Genes Immun 2009; 10(1): 68-76.
[http://dx.doi.org/10.1038/gene.2008.94] [PMID: 19092842]

[7]   Tzioufas AG, Kapsogeorgou EK, Moutsopoulos HM. Pathogenesis of Sjögren's syndrome: what we know and what we should learn. J Autoimmun 2012; 39(1-2): 4-8.
[http://dx.doi.org/10.1016/j.jaut.2012.01.002] [PMID: 22326205]

[8]   Katsifis GE, Moutsopoulos NM, Wahl SM. T lymphocytes in Sjögren's syndrome: contributors to and regulators of pathophysiology. Clin Rev Allergy Immunol 2007; 32(3): 252-64.
[http://dx.doi.org/10.1007/s12016-007-8011-8] [PMID: 17992592]

[9]   Mavragani CP, Moutsopoulos HM. Sjögren syndrome. CMAJ 2014; 186(15): E579-86.
[http://dx.doi.org/10.1503/cmaj.122037] [PMID: 24566651]

[10]   Theander E, Vasaitis L, Baecklund E, *et al.* Lymphoid organisation in labial salivary gland biopsies is a possible predictor for the development of malignant lymphoma in primary Sjögren's syndrome. Ann Rheum Dis 2011; 70(8): 1363-8.
[http://dx.doi.org/10.1136/ard.2010.144782] [PMID: 21715359]

[11]   Mavragani CP, Fragoulis GE, Moutsopoulos HM. Endocrine alterations in primary Sjogren's syndrome: an overview. J Autoimmun 2012; 39(4): 354-8.
[http://dx.doi.org/10.1016/j.jaut.2012.05.011] [PMID: 22695186]

[12]   Barone F, Bombardieri M, Manzo A, *et al.* Association of CXCL13 and CCL21 expression with the progressive organization of lymphoid-like structures in Sjögren's syndrome. Arthritis Rheum 2005; 52(6): 1773-84.
[http://dx.doi.org/10.1002/art.21062] [PMID: 15934082]

[13]   Wahren-Herlenius M, Dörner T. Immunopathogenic mechanisms of systemic autoimmune disease. Lancet 2013; 382(9894): 819-31.
[http://dx.doi.org/10.1016/S0140-6736(13)60954-X] [PMID: 23993191]

[14]   Kyriakidis NC, Kapsogeorgou EK, Tzioufas AG. A comprehensive review of autoantibodies in primary Sjögren's syndrome: clinical phenotypes and regulatory mechanisms. J Autoimmun 2014; 51: 67-74.
[http://dx.doi.org/10.1016/j.jaut.2013.11.001] [PMID: 24333103]

[15]   Fisher BA, Brown RM, Bowman SJ, Barone F. A review of salivary gland histopathology in primary Sjögren's syndrome with a focus on its potential as a clinical trials biomarker. Ann Rheum Dis 2015; 74(9): 1645-50.
[http://dx.doi.org/10.1136/annrheumdis-2015-207499] [PMID: 26034044]

[16]   Greenspan JS, Daniels TE, Talal N, Sylvester RA. The histopathology of Sjögren's syndrome in labial salivary gland biopsies. Oral Surg Oral Med Oral Pathol 1974; 37(2): 217-29.
[http://dx.doi.org/10.1016/0030-4220(74)90417-4] [PMID: 4589360]

[17]   Fisher BA, Jonsson R, Daniels T, *et al.* Standardisation of labial salivary gland histopathology in clinical trials in primary Sjögren's syndrome. Ann Rheum Dis 2017; 76(7): 1161-8.
[http://dx.doi.org/10.1136/annrheumdis-2016-210448] [PMID: 27965259]

[18]   Vitali C, Bombardieri S, Jonsson R, *et al.* Classification criteria for Sjögren's syndrome: a revised version of the European criteria proposed by the American-European Consensus Group. Ann Rheum Dis 2002; 61(6): 554-8.
[http://dx.doi.org/10.1136/ard.61.6.554] [PMID: 12006334]

[19]   Vitali C, Bombardieri S, Moutsopoulos HM, *et al.* Preliminary classification criteria for Sjögren's syndrome. Results of a prospective concerted action supported by the European Community. Arthritis Rheum 1993; 36: 340-7.
[http://dx.doi.org/10.1002/art.1780360309] [PMID: 8452579]

[20]   Ramos-Casals M, Tzioufas AG, Stone JH, Sisó A, Bosch X. Treatment of primary Sjögren syndrome: a systematic review. JAMA 2010; 304(4): 452-60.
[http://dx.doi.org/10.1001/jama.2010.1014] [PMID: 20664046]

[21]   Pinto A. Management of xerostomia and other complications of Sjögren's syndrome. Oral Maxillofac Surg Clin North Am 2014; 26(1): 63-73.
[http://dx.doi.org/10.1016/j.coms.2013.09.010] [PMID: 24287194]

[22]   Ramos-Casals M, Tzioufas AG, Font J. Primary Sjögren's syndrome: new clinical and therapeutic concepts. Ann Rheum Dis 2005; 64(3): 347-54.
[http://dx.doi.org/10.1136/ard.2004.025676] [PMID: 15498797]

[23]   Westhoff G, Dörner T, Zink A. Fatigue and depression predict physician visits and work disability in women with primary Sjögren's syndrome: results from a cohort study. Rheumatology (Oxford) 2012; 51(2): 262-9.
[http://dx.doi.org/10.1093/rheumatology/ker208] [PMID: 21705778]

[24]   Fauchais AL, Ouattara B, Gondran G, *et al.* Articular manifestations in primary Sjögren's syndrome: clinical significance and prognosis of 188 patients. Rheumatology (Oxford) 2010; 49(6): 1164-72.
[http://dx.doi.org/10.1093/rheumatology/keq047] [PMID: 20299380]

[25]   Brito-Zerón P, Retamozo S, Akasbi M, *et al.* Annular erythema in primary Sjogren's syndrome: description of 43 non-Asian cases. Lupus 2014; 23(2): 166-75.
[http://dx.doi.org/10.1177/0961203313515764] [PMID: 24326481]

[26]   Vassiliou VA, Moyssakis I, Boki KA, Moutsopoulos HM. Is the heart affected in primary Sjögren's syndrome? An echocardiographic study. Clin Exp Rheumatol 2008; 26(1): 109-12.
[PMID: 18328155]

[27]   Liang D, Lu J, Guo A. Sjögren's syndrome accompanied with interstitial cystitis: a case report and review of the literature. Clin Rheumatol 2014; 33(8): 1189-93.
[http://dx.doi.org/10.1007/s10067-013-2480-3] [PMID: 24395198]

[28]   Brito-Zerón P, Akasbi M, Bosch X, *et al.* Classification and characterisation of peripheral neuropathies in 102 patients with primary Sjögren's syndrome. Clin Exp Rheumatol 2013; 31(1): 103-10.
[PMID: 23020902]

[29]   Ashraf VV, Bhasi R, Kumar RP, Girija AS. Primary Sjögren's syndrome manifesting as multiple cranial neuropathies: MRI findings. Ann Indian Acad Neurol 2009; 12(2): 124-6.
[http://dx.doi.org/10.4103/0972-2327.53083] [PMID: 20142860]

[30]   Rossi R, Valeria Saddi M. Subacute aseptic meningitis as neurological manifestation of primary Sjögren's syndrome. Clin Neurol Neurosurg 2006; 108(7): 688-91.

[http://dx.doi.org/10.1016/j.clineuro.2005.05.015] [PMID: 16054750]

[31]   Voulgarelis M, Tzioufas AG. Current aspects of pathogenesis of Sjögren's syndrome. Ther Adv Musculoskelet Dis 2010; 2(6): 325-34.
[http://dx.doi.org/10.1177/1759720X10381431] [PMID: 22870458]

[32]   Ramos-Casals M, Stone JH, Cid MC, Bosch X. The cryoglobulinaemias. Lancet 2012; 379(9813): 348-60.
[http://dx.doi.org/10.1016/S0140-6736(11)60242-0] [PMID: 21868085]

[33]   Retamozo S, Akasbi M, Brito-Zerón P, *et al.* Anti-Ro52 antibody testing influences the classification and clinical characterisation of primary Sjögren's syndrome. Clin Exp Rheumatol 2012; 30(5): 686-92.
[PMID: 22704838]

[34]   Routsias JG, Tzioufas AG. B-cell epitopes of the intracellular autoantigens Ro/SSA and La/SSB: tools to study the regulation of the autoimmune response. J Autoimmun 2010; 35(3): 256-64.
[http://dx.doi.org/10.1016/j.jaut.2010.06.016] [PMID: 20643529]

[35]   Voulgarelis M, Ziakas PD, Papageorgiou A, Baimpa E, Tzioufas AG, Moutsopoulos HM. Prognosis and outcome of non-Hodgkin lymphoma in primary Sjögren syndrome. Medicine (Baltimore) 2012; 91(1): 1-9.
[http://dx.doi.org/10.1097/MD.0b013e31824125e4] [PMID: 22198497]

[36]   Seror R, Ravaud P, Bowman SJ, *et al.* EULAR Sjogren's syndrome disease activity index: development of a consensus systemic disease activity index for primary Sjogren's syndrome. Ann Rheum Dis 2010; 69(6): 1103-9.
[http://dx.doi.org/10.1136/ard.2009.110619] [PMID: 19561361]

[37]   Seror R, Ravaud P, Mariette X, *et al.* EULAR Sjogren's Syndrome Patient Reported Index (ESSPRI): development of a consensus patient index for primary Sjogren's syndrome. Ann Rheum Dis 2011; 70(6): 968-72.
[http://dx.doi.org/10.1136/ard.2010.143743] [PMID: 21345815]

[38]   Gottenberg JE, Guillevin L, Lambotte O, *et al.* Tolerance and short term efficacy of rituximab in 43 patients with systemic autoimmune diseases. Ann Rheum Dis 2005; 64(6): 913-20.
[http://dx.doi.org/10.1136/ard.2004.029694] [PMID: 15550531]

[39]   Masaki Y, Dong L, Kurose N, *et al.* Proposal for a new clinical entity, IgG4-positive multiorgan lymphoproliferative syndrome: analysis of 64 cases of IgG4-related disorders. Ann Rheum Dis 2009; 68(8): 1310-5.
[http://dx.doi.org/10.1136/ard.2008.089169] [PMID: 18701557]

CHAPTER 6

Polymyositis and Dermatomyositis

Abstract: Dermatomyositis and polymyositis are inflammatory myopathies with muscle inflammation and proximal muscle weakness. Skin examination, muscle enzyme measurement (creatinine kinase, aldolase) assessment of antinuclear and myositis-specific antibodies (MSA), muscle or skin biopsy, electromyography (EMG), magnetic resonance imaging (MRI) of skeletal muscle and exclusion of malignancy are very important.

Histologic signs of DM and PM include degeneration, regeneration, inflammatory cell infiltration and ultimately, muscle fiber necrosis. In DM, the cellular infiltrate is perifascicular and perivascular with infiltration of B lymphocytes and plasmacytoid dendritic cells. In PM, the cellular infiltrate in muscle is in the fascicle, with cytotoxic CD8+ T cells. Skin changes characteristic of DM are Gottron's papules, a heliotrope rash and V sign. EMG findings include spontaneous fibrillations, positive sharp waves, and complex repetitive discharges.

DM is diagnosed in patients with symmetrical proximal muscle weakness, increased muscle enzymes and a specific rash. Biopsy is not required.

EMG and muscle biopsy may be useful in patients who have atypical findings to exclude other diseases such as inclusion body myositis (IBM), metabolic myopathy, or muscle dystrophies.

Exclusion of other diseases such as inflammatory myopathies, motor neuron disease, myasthenia gravis, muscular dystrophies, inherited, metabolic, drug-induced, endocrine, and infectious myopathies must be performed.

Muscle strength and CK levels monitor disease activity. GCS are the main lines of treatment used. Combined therapy includes methotrexate, azathioprine and antimalarial drugs.

Cyclophospamide and intravenous gamma-globulin have a role in life-threatening cases. Plasmapheresis is used only when the above mentioned therapies have failed.

Keywords: Aldolase, ANA, Creatinine kinase, Dermatomyositis, Drug-induced, Electromyography (EMG), Endocrine myopathies, Idiopathic inflammatory myopathies, Inherited, Malignancy, Metabolic, Motor neuron disease, MRI, Muscle biopsy, Muscle enzyme, Muscle fiber necrosis, Muscle weakness,

Muscular dystrophies, Myasthenia gravis, Myositis-specific antibodies (MSA), Polymyositis, Skin biopsy.

INTRODUCTION

Idiopathic inflammatory myopathies (IIMs) are diseases involving muscles with chronic and progressive symmetrical proximal muscle weakness. IIMs are isolated or include with muscular features and are connected with connective tissue diseases like SS, systemic sclerosis, MCTD, SLE or RA. IIMs is classified into six types: dermatomyositis (DM), juvenile dermatomyositis (JDM), clinically amyopathic dermatomyositis (CADM), polymyositis (PM), inclusion body myositis (IDM) and immune mediated necrotizing myopathy (IMNM). Others types include necrotizing myositis, chronic granulomatous myositis associated with sarcoidosis, orbital myositis, focal myositis and eosinophilic myositis.

Polymyositis is chronic inflammation of striated muscle (myositis) with characteristic dermatological features (rash of dermatomyositis) and different systemic complications. Patients with DM and PM differ from patients with systemic rheumatic diseases, patients with metabolic, infections, malignant disorders, neuropathies, neuromuscular diseases, and other myopathies, including drug-induced myopathy, only after examination.

IIMs are confirmed by the presence of myositis –specific and myositis-associated autoantibodies (MSAs/MAAs) [1].

EPIDEMIOLOGY

IIMs affect adults and children, and there is a 2:1 female predisposition. The incidence per year is 2 – 7 cases per million inhibitans. The disease occurs mostly at the age of 50-60 years, although PM and DM may both start at any age. The incidence per year of IBM is about 1-2 per million adults and is more common in men [2].

ETIOPATHOGENESIS

Genetic Factors

IIM diseases susceptibility is linked to human leucocyte antigen (HLA) genes class II alleles. In Caucasians with HLA-DRB1*0301 and DQA1*0501 haplotypes there is a predisposition for the disease, but in Asians, HLA-B7 and DQA1*01 appear to have a protective association [3]. An increased association was found between subsets of myositis with autoantibody profiles like anti-Jo-1 and HLA-DRB1*0301 and DQA1*0501, and between anti-Mi-2 and DRB1*07 and DQA*0201 [3]. For IBM there is an association with HLA-DRB1*0301,DRB*0101, DQB1*0201 and DRw52 [3].

The associations are between myositis and non-HLA genes, like those for proinflammatory cytokines (-308TNFA genotype) [4, 5].

Another non-MHC single-nucleotide polymorphism associated with myositis is linked to the *PTPN22* gene [4, 5].

Environmental Factors

Viral infections such as Coxsackie, echo, influenza and retrovirus infections may contribute to the onset of IIM. Other factors include exposure to UV light and vitamin D deficiency.

Exposure to UV light predisposes to the development of the subset with Mi-2 autoantibodies.

Vitamin D deficiency is a risk factor for all IIM subtypes, including the anti-Jo-1 antibodies association [6].

The most common drug-induced myopathy is caused by statins. Others include fibrates and nicotinic acid. Muscle biopsy samples in statin-induced myopathy are usually normal without inflammatory cell infiltrates. In more severe cases myonecrosis of fibres may be seen with or without inflammatory cell infiltration however the prognosis is good [7].

The mechanism of drug-involved myopathies is unknown. Statins, inhibitors of 3-hydroxy-3-methylglutaryl-CoA (HGM-CoA) reductase (HMGCR), and this inhibition may interfere with energy production, leading to damage of muscle fiber and the overexpression of HMGCR by regenerating muscle fibers and development of anti-HMGCR antibodies [8]. This is strongly associated with the HLA-DRB1*1101 gene, and suggests an autoimmune origin [8].

Other drugs that may induce myopathies are cimetidine, antimalarials, colchicines, penicillamine, antipsychotics, cocaine, certain antiretrovirals.

Alcohol may induce a myopathy and accumulation of fat in muscle fibres without the presence of inflammation, as well as GCS, which is not associated with characteristic histopathological changes, but shows a non-specific type II fibre atrophy.

PATHOGENESIS

T lymphocytes and macrophages are the main cells in the inflammation in IIM, with higher CD8 T cell count than CD4 T cells in the endomysial infiltrates [9]. These infiltrates surround and invade fibers with non-necrotic muscle fibers. The inflammatory infiltrates of DM typically include CD4 T cells and macrophages, with a perivascular localization mainly in the perimysium [9]. CD28 null T cells secrete large amounts of inflammatory cytokines and cytotoxic molecules – granzymes and perforins [10]. IL17 can trigger the release of a number of proinflammatory TH1 cytokines IL-2, IL-1, IL-6 and IL-15 and can induce an increase in MHC I expression on muscle fibres [9].

B cells are found rarely in inflammatory infiltrates in IIM and they have a perivascular localization in DM infiltrates, particularly in the subtype associated with calcinosis in children [9].

The increase of tissue-specific antigen immunogenicity is due to increase levels of antigen expression in muscle tissue and increased activity of adjuvant antigens [10].

Activation of IFN alpha/beta pathways induce and maintain autoimmunity in IIM by increasing the maturation of B cells and DCs and stimulate production of IL-1-alpha, IL-1beta and TNFalpha [11].

Patient Interview

Patients history should include the severity, onset, duration, and distribution of muscle weakness. Patients history should include asking about difficulty in climbing stairs, getting up from a chair, and carrying heavy loads. Muscle weakness should be differentiated from cardiovascular or pulmonary symptoms like fatigue or shortness of breath on exertion, and from joint disease symptoms like limitation of movement and arthralgia.

Patients history should include the presence of dysphagia, which suggests esophageal involvement, and cough or shortness of breath due to pulmonary involvement. Patients should also be asked about any skin changes, photosensitivity, Raynaud phenomenon, and other symptoms. They should be asked if they have any symptoms suggesting malignancy, and should be ask about the using drugs that may cause myopathy, particularly statins.

Physical Examination

Importantly, examination should be focused on skin, muscles, and joints. The skin of the scalp, face, eyelids, hands, fingers should be carefully examined. A general physical examination is important and should focus on the heart and lungs. A joint examination should be performed to detect inflammation. A neurological and neuromuscular examination is also important to confirm the severity and extent of weakness and muscle tenderness, and to investigate for any abnormal neurological findings.

Laboratory Examinations

Laboratory examinations of muscle enzymes (creatinine kinase and aldolase), a complete blood count with differential, creatinine, erythrocyte sedimentation rate (ESR), C-reactive protein (CRP), liver function tests, and thyroid-stimulating hormone (TSH) should be measured.

Testing for antinuclear antibodies (ANA); anti-Ro/SSA, anti-La/SSB, anti-ribonucleoprotein (RNP), anti-Sm; and myositis-associated and myositis-specific antibodies including anti-Jo-1 and other anti-synthetase antibodies, as well as antibodies directed against the Mi2, SRP, PM/Scl, and Ku antigens, should be performed [11].

It is crucial to investigate for defects in carbohydrate, lipid, or purine metabolism to detect metabolic myopathies.

Abnormal proteins in immunohistological assays include:

Dystrophin for Duchenne/Becker dystrophy.

Merosin for congenital muscular dystrophy.

Sarcoglycan for limb-girdle muscular dystrophy.

IMAGING

Chest radiographs show the presence of pulmonary involvement, such as interstitial lung disease, especially in patients with an antisynthetase syndrome. In patients with pulmonary symptoms or with abnormal chest radiographs showing interstitial lung disease, CT and pulmonary function tests must be performed. Association of dermatomyositis with malignancy in middle-aged and elderly population is observed in half of patients [12].

MUSCLE BIOPSY

Histopathological changes differentiated DM and PM from each other and from other myopathies.

DM and PM histological examinations show degeneration, regeneration, inflammatory cell infiltrate and muscle fiber necrosis [9].

DM in histopathological exams is characterized by injury to capillaries, perifascicular myofibers, perifascicular atrophy and fibrosis. The main inflammatory infiltrate is in the perimysial region with CD4+ cells, macrophages and B cells. Pathological muscle fibers seen in one part of the fascicle suggest microinfarct due to dysfunction of blood vessel [9]. The terminal complement C5b-9 membrane attack complex is often present in vessel walls.

PM is characterized in histopathological studies by cellular infiltrations in the fascicle, with inflammatory cells in individual muscle fibers. Necrotic and regenerating muscle fibers are scattered throughout the fascicle. Muscle fiber size varies. There are no signs of vasculopathy or immune complex deposition [9]. Myofiber injury is a consequence of CD8+ cytotoxic T lymphocytes in myofibers. The inflammation of perivascular, perimysial, or endomysial regions with infiltration of macrophages, dendritic cells, plasma cells is observed. Increased expression of class I major histocompatibility complex antigens by the muscle fibers is present [9].

Autoimmune necrotizing myopathy presents with scattered necrotic muscle fibers without perifascicular atrophy [8].

The biopsy should be taken from a muscle that on physical examination is weak but not atrophied. Muscle biopsy is usually performed on the quadriceps or the deltoid. Muscles with severe weakness and atrophy, or recent EMG testing are not used and biopsy of the calf muscles is not performed due to findings of artefacts.

SKIN BIOPSY

Patients with DM must have a skin biopsy.

In light microscopy, DM skin changes include atrophy of the epidermis with vacuolar changes in the basal keratinocyte layer, and a perivascular lymphocytic infiltrate in the dermis [13]. Patients with DM often have increased dermal mucin.

Direct immunofluorescence shows deposition of complement proteins and immunoglobulin at the dermal-epidermal junction. Deposits of the membrane attack complex are along the dermal-epidermal junction and within the walls of dermal blood vessels [14].

A 4 mm punch biopsy sample should be used for histological examination on light microscopy with hematoxylin and eosin staining.

ELECTROMYOGRAPHY

EMG differentatiates myopathy weakness from neuropathic disorders, for example, as in amyotrophic lateral sclerosis, peripheral polyneuropathy or myasthenia gravis.

EMG shows increased insertional activity and spontaneous fibrillations, abnormal myopathic low-amplitude, short-duration polyphasic motor unit potential and complex repetitive discharges.

An increased number of motor units firing rapidly is an early finding in myopathy causing a low level of contraction. Insertional activity, fibrillation potentials, and complex repetitive discharges can be seen in inflammatory myopathies.

MAGNETIC RESONANCE IMAGING (MRI)

MRI may reveal areas of increased T2 signal in muscles to better select a biopsy location [15].

MRI of skeletal muscles is a non-invasive test used to evaluate patients with myopathy and show areas of muscle inflammation, edema with active myositis, fibrosis, and calcification. It may also assess large areas of muscle, and is therefore needed to differentiate nonspecific changes that occur in rhabdomyolysis, muscular dystrophy, or metabolic myopathy [15].

DIAGNOSIS

Several groups of classification criteria have been used for dermatomyositis and polymyositis to define these disorders for clinical and epidemiologic research. The mostly commonly used classification criteria developed by Bohan and Peter [16, 17] in 1975 have been used for several decades.

Bohan and Peter criteria for diagnosis of polymyositis and dermatomyositis are [16, 17]:

1. Symmetrical proximal muscle weakness

2. Muscle biopsy evidence of myositis

3. Elevated serum muscle enzymes

4. Characteristic electromyographic pattern

5. Typical rash of dermatomyositis.

Diagnostic criteria polymyositis: definite: all of 1-4, probable: any 3 of 1-4, possible: any 2 of 1-4.

Diagnostic criteria dermatomyositis: definite: 5 plus any 3 of 1-4, probable: 5 plus any 2 of 1-4, possible: 5 plus any 1 of 1-4.

Patients with skin changes and at least three of the other four criteria met the requirements for definite DM according to these criteria, while requirements for definite PM were met by those with all four criteria other than the cutaneous features [16, 17]. Patients with disorders that may present similarly were excluded. Those disorders included central or peripheral neurologic disease; muscular dystrophy; granulomatous myositis, such as sarcoidosis; infectious muscle disease (*e.g.* trichinosis or toxoplasmosis); recent exposure to myopathic drugs or toxins; rhabdomyolysis, metabolic muscle disease; myopathic endocrinopathy; and myasthenia gravis. Patients who did not have any of the exclusions and did not meet these criteria are diagnosed with possible or probable DM or PM, depending upon the number of criteria met [16, 17].

A tissue biopsy is not needed to confirm the diagnosis of DM in patients with symmetric proximal muscle weakness and a marked elevation of muscle enzymes, and where there is no other probable diagnosis. These include patients with cutaneous changes (Gottron's papules or a heliotrop eruption) or patients with the antisynthetase syndrome (rash, polyarthritis, Raynaud phenomenon, interstitial lung disease, and presence of anti-Jo-1 antibodies) [6].

Patients with DM or PM with typical but nonspecific symptoms of symmetric proximal muscle weakness and elevated muscle enzymes, in the absence of specific cutaneous manifestations or myositis-specific antibodies (MSA) need tissue muscle biopsy for confirmation.

In patients with atypical presentations, to be able to differentiate between myopathic and neuropathic disorders causing weakness, an EMG and/or MRI should be undertaken. After these examinations, patients with a suspicion of myopathy should have a muscle biopsy to confirm the diagnosis of DM or PM and to exclude other diseases, such as inclusion body myositis (IBM), metabolic or mitochondrial myopathy, muscular dystrophy, necrotizing myositis, or drug-induced myopathy. Atypical symptoms that suggest another diagnosis are asymmetrical or distal weakness, intermittent symptoms, painful muscles, big muscle atrophy, family history of muscle disease, a history of drugs sometimes associated with myopathy, neuropathic symptoms.

Pathognomonic signs in dermatomyositis are Gottron's papules (60-80% of patients), heliotrop rash (50% or fewer) and less specific signs in dermatomyositis: photosensitivity, "V sign" over the anterior chest, calcinosis, "mechanic's hands", scleromyxedema, vitiligo, poikiloderma.

IMPORTANT DISEASE ASSESSMENT

Malignancy

Patients with DM or PM should have a physical examination with breast, rectal, and gynecological exam, laboratory testing; and cancer screening tests (*e.g.*, mammography, gastroscopy, colonoscopy, chest and abdominal CT).

Cardiac Involvement

Patients with cardiac muscle involvement, including symptoms of heart failure or of conduction abnormalities, an echocardiogram and electrocardiogram must be undertaken [18].

Pulmonary Disease

Patients with pulmonary symptoms *e.g.*, dyspnea or cough or with abnormalities on physical examination or on plain radiography of the chest, pulmonary function testing and computed tomography (CT) of the chest should be performed.

Esophageal Dysfunction

Patients with esophageal dysmotility, and symptoms of dysphagia or suspicion of aspiration pneumonia should have esophageal motility testing.

NON-NEUROMUSCULAR CAUSES OF WEAKNESS

EPISODIC WEAKNESS: hypotension, cardiac arrhythmias, hypoxia, hypercapnia, hyperventilation, hypoglycemia, cerebrovascular insufficiency, emotional states (hyperventilation, anxiety).

PERSISTENT WEAKNESS: anemia, chronic or acute infections, malignancy, malnutrition, advanced organ system failure (lung, heart, liver, kidney), metabolic disorders (hyperthyroidism, hyperparathyroidism, hypophosphatemia).

Differential diagnosis of muscle weakness: denervate conditions, genetic muscular dystrophies, myositis ossificans, endocrine myopathies, metabolic myopathies, toxic myopathies, carcinomatous myopathies, acute rhabdomyolysis, polymyalgia rheumatic [19].

The differential diagnosis of DM and PM include: other inflammatory myopathies, motor neuron disease, myasthenia gra vis, muscular dystrophies, and inherited, metabolic, drug-induced, endocrine, and infectious myopathies [19].

CLINICALLY AMYOPATHIC DERMATOMYOSITIS (CADM)

Clinically amyopathic dermatomyositis is a clinically distinct subgroup of dermatomyositis characterized by unique dermatological manifestations without muscle involvement. Some of the skin changes that suggest dermatomyositis include a pink rash on the face, neck, forearms and upper chest; Gottron's papules and heliotrope eyelids. Clinically amyopathic dermatomyositis is frequently associated with interstitial lung disease, which usually has a rapidly progressive, fatal clinical course. Some cases have been associated with internal malignancy. Treatment may include sun avoidance, topical GCS, antimalarial agents, MTX, MMF, or intravenous immunoglobulin.

INCLUSION BODY MYOSITIS (IBM)

Proximal muscle weakness that is painless and symmetrical, which may include a rash, increase in serum muscle enzymes (CK), abnormal electromyogram and muscle biopsy, that shows inflammatory infiltrates, involvement of other organ systems including the lung, heart, gastrointestinal tract and joints is characteristic for IBM. IBM is an inflammatory myopathy with a more severe onset and distal muscle weakness that is less serious than in PM. Asymmetric muscle atrophy and weakness of the wrist and finger flexor in the upper extremities with weakness of the quadriceps and anterior muscles in the legs is very characteristic.

In IBM serum muscle enzyme levels are 10 times lower than in PM and the presence of typical inclusion bodies on muscle biopsy is pathognomonic [20]. MRI findings are changes along fascial planes in PM, but in IBM changes throughout the muscle [21]. Fatty infiltration and muscle atrophy are seen often in IBM than in PM [21].

IMMUNE MEDIATED DRUG-INDUCED MYOPATHY (IMNM)

Drugs such as glucocortiocoids, statins [7], antimalarials, antipsychotics, colchicines, penicillamine, alcohol, cocaine, and certain antiretrovirals result in myopathy similar to the inflammatory myopathies. Electromyography (EMG) and muscle biopsy helps in differentiating drug-induced myopathy.

NECROTIZING MYOPATHY

Autoimmune necrotizing myopathy mimics PM with proximal upper and lower extremity muscle weakness, but is different histologically from PM or DM due to presence of necrotic muscle fibers without significant inflammatory cell infiltrate around non-necrotic fibers, and a lack of perifascicular atrophy [9]. It may occur after exposure to statins, but, unlike statin-induced myopathy, it remains after withdrawal of the drug [22].

In some patients it is observed the presence of antibodies to signal recognition peptides or to antibodies anti 200/100 [23], which are present in patients with statin-induced necrotizing myopathy and recognizes the hydroxymethylglutaryl (HMG)-coenzyme A reductase protein [8].

HYPOTHYROIDISM

Myopathy with hypothyroidism has a subacute onset of proximal muscle weakness and elevated muscle enzymes. Clinical symptoms of hypothyroidism are delayed relaxation phase of the deep tendon reflexes, lack of fibrillation potentials on electromyogram with normal motor units, and the absence of inflammatory infiltrations on muscle biopsy, differentiate hypothyroid myopathy from polymyositis. Screening test includes thyroid-stimulating hormone (TSH) measurement.

HIV INFECTION

Human immunodeficiency virus (HIV) infections is often associated with an inflammatory myopathy in the early and later stages of infection. It became much less common after the advent of HAART therapy [24]. Patients with HIV myopathy have myalgias and muscle tenderness with elevated muscle enzymes. EMG in HIV myopathy is similar to PM; muscle biopsy shows an endomysial mononuclear cell infiltrate with lesser accumulation of inflammatory cells (mostly CD8 T cells and macrophages) around vessels or in the interfascicular space.

HIV myopathy has a better prognosis than PM. For some patients without improvement, high-dose steroids are recommended [25] and methotrexate and azathioprine must be used with caution [25].

In HIV-infected patients with myopathy, rhabdomyolysis and opportunistic infections (*e.g.*, toxoplasmosis), should be excluded.

MYASTHENIA GRAVIS

Myasthenia gravis is a disease of the neuromuscular junction, caused by antibodies to the acetylocholine receptor. In myasthenia gravis it there is muscle fatigability and muscle weakness increases with exercise. Diffuse weakness appears without symptoms of fatigue. Myasthenia gravis is differentiated from PM by the presence of facial muscle weakness, normal muscle enzymes, characteristic EMG changes, and anti-acetylocholine receptor antibodies.

MUSCLE DYSTROPHY

The muscular dystrophies are progressive myopathic disorders caused by defects in genes for normal muscle function. The inflammatory cell infiltrate in muscular dystrophy is only in areas in proximity to necrotic muscle fibers.

OTHER MUSCLE DISEASES

Other myopathies that may be similar to PM are acute myopathy after acute viral or bacterial infections (pyomyositis), immobilization, and trauma. The disease course is acute with fulminant symptoms often complicated by rhabdomyolysis.

Chronic graft-versus-host disease (GVHD) with muscle disease is clinically and histopathologically similar to PM [26]. The onset of this myositis is more than one year after transplantation [27]. The frequency is 0.6% [27].

Amyloid myopathy occurs in immunoglobulin-related or familial amyloidosis [28].

Sarcoid myopathy occurs in patients with sarcoidosis, is asymptomatic and has clinical and histological manifestations of sarcoidosis.

Parasitic infections, *e.g.* trichinellosis, cause muscle pain, eosinophilia and elevated muscle enzymes after consuming inadequately cooked meat. Muscle biopsy confirms the diagnosis.

Diabetic myopathy and diabetic muscle infarction are characterized by acute onset of pain with weakness of the proximal leg and autonomic failure. The diagnosis of diabetic muscle infarction is clinical, with a history of acute or subacute muscle pain, swelling, and tenderness, in the muscles of the thigh and calf.

Other Skin Diseases

Patients with systemic lupus erythematosus (SLE) may develop cutaneous lesions like facial erythema and other photosensitive eruptions, resembling some of the facial changes seen in DM. However, the midfacial erythematous eruption in DM often does not spare the nasolabial folds.

Scalp involvement in psoriasis or seborrheic dermatitis may be similar to scalp DM, but a thicker, silvery or micaceous scaling may be present in psoriasis, and a more yellow, greasy scaling may be seen in seborrheic dermatitis. Scalp DM may be differentiated from both of these disorders on skin biopsy by showing characteristic vacuolar interface changes.

SERUM AUTOANTIBODIES [9]

Myositis Specific Antibodies (MSA)
Jo-1 antibodies
No Jo-1: PL-7, PL-12, EJ,OJ, KS
Not antisynthetase antibodies
MJ, SRP, MDA5, TIF-1y, SAE, Mi-2
Myositis Associated Antibodies (MAA):
PM-Scl, U1-RNP, Ku, SSA
PM-Scl – 10% – overlap with SS
U1-RNP – 10% – MCTD
Mi-2 – 10% – DM, SRP <5% – antisynthetase syndrome
EJ, OJ, KS, PMS-1, Ku 5% – overlap with SS [9].

MANAGEMENT OF INFLAMMATORY MUSCLE DISEASE

Biopsy is the gold standard procedure used to identify non-responding myopathies such as inclusion body myositis. Muscle strength and CK levels are used most frequently to assess disease activity and therapy efficacy. GCS are the treatment of choice.

Drugs most frequently used for combined therapy are methotrexate, azathioprine and antimalarial drugs.

Cyclophospamide and/or intravenous gamma-globulin may have an important effect in some life-threatening cases.

Ciclosporin, mofetil mycophenolate may also have a role in non-responding cases.

Plasmapheresis is reserved if the above mentioned therapies fail.

Treatment of inclusion body myositis remains unsatisfactory.

Biological drugs have not established a role in PM and DM. Rituximab may be useful for PM and DM, but further trials are needed. Other drugs include the IL-1 receptor antagonist, eculizumab, and the monoclonal antibodies against the C5 complement component and INFß, but randomized trials are needed.

REFERENCES

[1]   Troyanov Y, Targoff IN, Tremblay JL, Goulet JR, Raymond Y, Senécal JL. Novel classification of idiopathic inflammatory myopathies based on overlap syndrome features and autoantibodies: analysis of 100 French Canadian patients. Medicine (Baltimore) 2005; 84(4): 231-49.
[http://dx.doi.org/10.1097/01.md.0000173991.74008.b0] [PMID: 16010208]

[2]   Bernatsky S, Joseph L, Pineau CA, *et al.* Estimating the prevalence of polymyositis and dermatomyositis from administrative data: age, sex and regional differences. Ann Rheum Dis 2009; 68(7): 1192-6.
[http://dx.doi.org/10.1136/ard.2008.093161] [PMID: 18713785]

[3]   O'Hanlon TP, Carrick DM, Targoff IN, *et al.* Immunogenetic risk and protective factors for the idiopathic inflammatory myopathies: distinct HLA-A, -B, -Cw, -DRB1, and -DQA1 allelic profiles distinguish European American patients with different myositis autoantibodies. Medicine (Baltimore) 2006; 85(2): 111-27.
[http://dx.doi.org/10.1097/01.md.0000217525.82287.eb] [PMID: 16609350]

[4]   Greenberg SA. A gene expression approach to study perturbed pathways in myositis. Curr Opin Rheumatol 2007; 19(6): 536-41.
[http://dx.doi.org/10.1097/BOR.0b013e3282efe261] [PMID: 17917532]

[5]   Shamim EA, Rider LG, Pandey JP, *et al.* Differences in idiopathic inflammatory myopathy phenotypes and genotypes between Mesoamerican Mestizos and North American Caucasians: ethnogeographic influences in the genetics and clinical expression of myositis. Arthritis Rheum 2002; 46(7): 1885-93.
[http://dx.doi.org/10.1002/art.10358] [PMID: 12124873]

[6]   Stone KB, Oddis CV, Fertig N, *et al.* Anti-Jo-1 antibody levels correlate with disease activity in idiopathic inflammatory myopathy. Arthritis Rheum 2007; 56(9): 3125-31.
[http://dx.doi.org/10.1002/art.22865] [PMID: 17763431]

[7]   Padala S, Thompson PD. Statins as a possible cause of inflammatory and necrotizing myopathies. Atherosclerosis 2012; 222(1): 15-21.
[http://dx.doi.org/10.1016/j.atherosclerosis.2011.11.005] [PMID: 22154355]

[8]   Mammen AL, Chung T, Christopher-Stine L, *et al.* Autoantibodies against 3-hydroxy-3-methylglutaryl-coenzyme A reductase in patients with statin-associated autoimmune myopathy. Arthritis Rheum 2011; 63(3): 713-21.
[http://dx.doi.org/10.1002/art.30156] [PMID: 21360500]

[9]   Vattemi G, Mirabella M, Guglielmi V, *et al.* Muscle biopsy features of idiopathic inflammatory myopathies and differential diagnosis. Auto Immun Highlights 2014; 5(3): 77-85.
[http://dx.doi.org/10.1007/s13317-014-0062-2] [PMID: 26000159]

[10]   Suber TL, Casciola-Rosen L, Rosen A. Mechanisms of disease: autoantigens as clues to the pathogenesis of myositis. Nat Clin Pract Rheumatol 2008; 4(4): 201-9.
[http://dx.doi.org/10.1038/ncprheum0760] [PMID: 18319710]

[11]   Ghirardello A, Bassi N, Palma L, *et al.* Autoantibodies in polymyositis and dermatomyositis. Curr Rheumatol Rep 2013; 15(6): 335-48.
[http://dx.doi.org/10.1007/s11926-013-0335-1] [PMID: 23591825]

[12]   Chinoy H, Fertig N, Oddis CV, Ollier WE, Cooper RG. The diagnostic utility of myositis autoantibody testing for predicting the risk of cancer-associated myositis. Ann Rheum Dis 2007; 66(10): 1345-9.
[http://dx.doi.org/10.1136/ard.2006.068502] [PMID: 17392346]

[13]   Dourmishev LA, Wollina U. Dermatomyositis: immunopathologic study of skin lesions. Acta Dermatovenerol Alp Panonica Adriat 2006; 15(1): 45-51.
[PMID: 16850099]

[14]   Magro CM, Segal JP, Crowson AN, Chadwick P. The phenotypic profile of dermatomyositis and lupus erythematosus: a comparative analysis. J Cutan Pathol 2010; 37(6): 659-71.
[http://dx.doi.org/10.1111/j.1600-0560.2009.01443.x] [PMID: 19891658]

[15]   May DA, Disler DG, Jones EA, Balkissoon AA, Manaster BJ. Abnormal signal intensity in skeletal muscle at MR imaging: patterns, pearls, and pitfalls. Radiographics 2000; 20(Spec No): S295-315.
[http://dx.doi.org/10.1148/radiographics.20.suppl_1.g00oc18s295] [PMID: 11046180]

[16]   Bohan A, Peter JB. Polymyositis and dermatomyositis (first of two parts). N Engl J Med 1975; 292(7): 344-7.
       [http://dx.doi.org/10.1056/NEJM197502132920706] [PMID: 1090839]

[17]   Bohan A, Peter JB. Polymyositis and dermatomyositis (second of two parts). N Engl J Med 1975; 292(8): 403-7.
       [http://dx.doi.org/10.1056/NEJM197502202920807] [PMID: 1089199]

[18]   Danieli MG, Gelardi C, Guerra F, Cardinaletti P, Pedini V, Gabrielli A. Cardiac involvement in polymyositis and dermatomyositis. Autoimmun Rev 2016; 15(5): 462-5.
       [http://dx.doi.org/10.1016/j.autrev.2016.01.015] [PMID: 26826433]

[19]   Diagnosis and differential diagnosis of dermatomyositis and polymyositis in adults, published in UpToDate, Waltham, MA 2013. https://www.upToDate.com/contents/diagnosis-and-differential-diagnosis-of-dermatomyositis-and-polymyositis-in-adults

[20]   Amato AA, Gronseth GS, Jackson CE, *et al.* Inclusion body myositis: clinical and pathological boundaries. Ann Neurol 1996; 40(4): 581-6.
       [http://dx.doi.org/10.1002/ana.410400407] [PMID: 8871577]

[21]   Dion E, Cherin P, Payan C, *et al.* Magnetic resonance imaging criteria for distinguishing between inclusion body myositis and polymyositis. J Rheumatol 2002; 29(9): 1897-906.
       [PMID: 12233884]

[22]   Grable-Esposito P, Katzberg HD, Greenberg SA, Srinivasan J, Katz J, Amato AA. Immune-mediated necrotizing myopathy associated with statins. Muscle Nerve 2010; 41(2): 185-90.
       [PMID: 19813188]

[23]   Christopher-Stine L, Casciola-Rosen LA, Hong G, Chung T, Corse AM, Mammen AL. A novel autoantibody recognizing 200-kd and 100-kd proteins is associated with an immune-mediated necrotizing myopathy. Arthritis Rheum 2010; 62(9): 2757-66.
       [http://dx.doi.org/10.1002/art.27572] [PMID: 20496415]

[24]   Authier FJ, Chariot P, Gherardi RK. Skeletal muscle involvement in human immunodeficiency virus (HIV)-infected patients in the era of highly active antiretroviral therapy (HAART). Muscle Nerve 2005; 32(3): 247-60.
       [http://dx.doi.org/10.1002/mus.20338] [PMID: 15902690]

[25]   Reveille JD. The changing spectrum of rheumatic disease in human immunodeficiency virus infection. Semin Arthritis Rheum 2000; 30(3): 147-66.
       [http://dx.doi.org/10.1053/sarh.2000.16527] [PMID: 11124280]

[26]   Parker P, Chao NJ, Ben-Ezra J, *et al.* Polymyositis as a manifestation of chronic graft-versus-host disease. Medicine (Baltimore) 1996; 75(5): 279-85.
       [http://dx.doi.org/10.1097/00005792-199609000-00004] [PMID: 8862349]

[27]   Stevens AM, Sullivan KM, Nelson JL. Polymyositis as a manifestation of chronic graft-versus-host disease. Rheumatology (Oxford) 2003; 42(1): 34-9.
       [http://dx.doi.org/10.1093/rheumatology/keg025] [PMID: 12509610]

[28]   Mandl LA, Folkerth RD, Pick MA, Weinblatt ME, Gravallese EM. Amyloid myopathy masquerading as polymyositis. J Rheumatol 2000; 27(4): 949-52.
       [PMID: 10782821]

CHAPTER 7

Scleroderma

Abstract: Systemic sclerosis (SSc) is a connective tissue disease characterized by fibrosis of the skin and internal organs, changes in the microvasculature and in cellular and humoral immunity.

The types of disorders include: localized scleroderma (morphea, linear scleroderma, en coup de sabre) and systemic sclerosis (diffuse cutaneous systemic sclerosis [dsSSc], limited cutaneous systemic sclerosis [lcSSc] and systemic sclerosis sine scleroderma).

LcSSc is a milder form with slow progression of skin involvement and visceral complications after 10-15 years, but with serious pulmonary arterial hypertension. DsSSc has fast progression of skin sclerosis, from weeks to months, and includes injuries to organs such as the lung, heart and kidney, which may lead to organ failure.

The presence of ANA was found in more than 90% of patients with SSc, anti-Scl-70 antibodies in patients with dcSSc in 30-40%, anticentromere antibodies (ACA) in patients with lcSSc in 80-90%.

Fibrosis is the end-stage representation of SSc pathogenesis.

Severe forms of the disease and rapidly progressive diffuse SSc with pulmonary, cardiac, and renal involvement, are associated with very high mortality rates, estimated at 40-50% in 5 years. No treatment effective therapy exists to stop fibrosis and disease progression beside autologous haemopoietic stem cell transplantation (AHSCT). Cyclophospamide has moderate efficacy in patients with ILD. Methotrexate may be used for the treatment of arthritis. Oesophageal dysmotility and reflux are treated with promotility agents, and proton pump inhibitors. In PAH endothelin receptor antagonists, with PDE5 inhibitor and prostaglandins are used. The most important manifestation is scleroderma renal crisis and is now treated using ACE inhibitors.

Keywords: ACE inhibitors, AHSCT, ANA, Anticentromere antibodies (ACA), Anti-RNA polymerases II and III antibodies, Anti-Scl-70 antibodies, Calcinosis, CREST syndrome, Cyclophospamide, Diffuse cutaneous systemic sclerosis (dsSSc), Endothelin receptor antagonists, Fibrosis, Limited cutaneous systemic sclerosis (lcSSc), Localized scleroderma, Oesophageal dysmotility, PAH, PDE5 inhibitor, Prostaglandins, Proton pump inhibitors, Raynaud's phenomenon, Sclerodactyly, Systemic sclerosis (SSc), Teleangiectasis, TGFβ.

Małgorzata Wisłowska

INTRODUCTION

Systemic sclerosis (SSc) is a connective tissue disease characterized by fibrosis of the skin and internal organs, changes in the microvasculature and in cellular and humoral immunity.

Classification used since 1980 was renewed in 2013.

The American College of Rheumatology 1980 criteria for the classification of Systemic Sclerosis are [1]:

Major Criterion

Proximal diffuse (truncal) sclerosis (skin tightness, thickening, non-pitting induration).

Minor Criteria

Sclerodactyly (only fingers and/or toes)

Digital pitting scars or loss of substance of the digital finger pads (pulp loss)

Bilateral basilar pulmonary fibrosis

The patient should fulfill the major criterion or two of the three minor criteria.

Systemic sclerosis 2013 ACR/EULAR classification is presented in Table **1 [2].**

Table 1. Systemic sclerosis 2013 ACR/EULAR classification.

Item	Subitem (s)	Weight/score
Skin thickening of the fingers of both hands extending proximal to the metacarpophalangeal joints (sufficient criterion)	-	9
Skin thickening of the fingers (only count the higher score)	Puffy fingers Sclerodactyly of the fingers (distal to the metacarpophalangeal joints but proximal to the proximal interphalangeal joints)	2 4
Fingertip lesions (only count the higher score)	Digital tip ulcer Fingertip pitting scars	2 3
Teleangiectasia	-	2
Abnormal nail fold capillary	-	2
Pulmonary arterial hypertension and/or interstitial lung disease (maximum score is 2)	Pulmonary arterial hypertension Interstitial lung disease	2 2

(Table 1) contd.....

Item	Subitem (s)	Weight/score
Raynaud's phenomenon	-	3
SSc-related autoantibodies (anticentromere, antitopoisomerase I (anti-Sc-70), anti-RNA polymerase III) maximum score is 3	Anticentromere Anti-topoisimerase I Anti-RNA polymerase III	3

The criteria cannot be used in patients with skin thickening sparing the fingers or in patients who have a scleroderma-like disorder that is explained by another disease (*e.g.* nephrogenic sclerosing fibrosis, generalized morphea, eosinophilic fasciitis, scleroderma diabeticorum, scleromyxodema, erythromelalgia, porphyria, lichen sclerosis, graft-versus-host disease, diabetic cheiroarthropathy). The total score is obtained by adding the maximum score in each category. To diagnose SSc, a total score of ≥9 should be obtained.

The Spectrum of Disorders in Scleroderma

Localized Scleroderma

Morphea

Linear scleroderma

En coup de sabre.

Systemic sclerosis

Diffuse cutaneous systemic sclerosis (dsSSc)

Limited cutaneous systemic sclerosis (lcSSc)

Systemic sclerosis sine scleroderma.

Localized scleroderma involves the skin and subcutaneous tissues, while SSc affects skin and internal organs, but pathogenesis of both forms are similar.

Limited cutaneous systemic sclerosis (lcSSc) involves skin from hands and feet to the elbows and knees, while diffuse cutaneous systemic sclerosis (dsSSc) involve skin thickening proximal to the knees and elbows. Limited cutaneous systemic sclerosis is a milder form with slow progression of skin involvement and visceral involvement after 10-15 years, but with pulmonary arterial hypertension and gastrointestinal involvement with malabsorption. The diffuse cutaneous systemic sclerosis has rapid skin sclerosis, within weeks to months, and rapid internal organ involvement such as lungs, heart and kidneys leading to its failure.

Systemic sclerosis without scleroderma is a rare subtype of SSc. It is characterized as SSc without any skin involvement but with vascular and serological features of SSc.

CREST (calcinosis, Raynaud's phenomenon, oesophageal dysmotility, sclerodactyly, and teleangiectasis) syndrome is an old term used for lcSSc. This abreviation does not include life threatening complications such as pulmonary arterial hypertension, mid-gut disease and lung fibrosis.

Epidemiology Reported cases of scleroderma occurs 7 – 20 per 1 000 000 in the general population per year [3]. The prevalence and severity of disease is different in different racial and ethnic groups. The incidence of scleroderma is higher in females than in males (3:1), and is greater in younger age groups (7:1) and less in patients over 50 years of age (2:1) [4]. The average age of onset of disease is approximately 50 years [4]. Prevalence is approximately 1 in 10 000 and incidence rates are at about 1 in 100 000. They may vary in different populations, suggesting a role in genetic predisposition and/or exposure to environmental factors.

The Genetics of Systemic Sclerosis

The genes for SSc can be divided into three main groups: 1- the genes involved in fibrosis, 2 - the genes involved in the immune response and 3 - the genes involved in vascular effects [5].

Fibrosis is the last stage of SSc. The genes that encode extracellular matrix proteins and their regulators (growth factors, cytokines, *etc.*) are very important.

Transforming growth factor beta (TGFß) regulation by fibrillin 1 (*FBN1)* gene is the main mediator in the process of fibrosis in SSc. Interactions between cells and the extracellular matrix are driven by the protein SPARC or osteonectin. TGFß and connective tissue growth factor may also contribute to the pathogenesis of SSc.

Caveolin-1 (CAV1) is the primary structural component of specialized plasma membrane microdomains called caveolae, which is an important inhibitor of tissue fibrosis that serves as a central molecule in transmembrane protein turnover and intracellular signaling cascades. It is a scaffolding protein that binds to different membrane receptors, G proteins and kinases, and regulates their activity. Within caveolae, *CAV1* is found next to cell membrane receptors for profibrotic mediators such as TGFß and platelet-derived growth factor. *CAV1* takes part in the pathogenesis of fibrosis by regulating of TGFß receptor internalization and degradation, decreasing TGFß signaling, and resulting in antifibrotic effects.

Genotype/protein expression correlations showed that the rs959173C protective allele was associated with increased *CAV1* protein expression [6].

Immune Response

SSc is associated with class II HLA molecules and genotypic variation that have been found between ethnic groups. A study of HLA class II genes (*DRB1, DQB1, DQA1, DPB1*) showed that the strongest associations were with the *DRB1*1104, DQA1*0501* and *DQB1*0301* haplotypes and the *DQB1* allele [7].

The *IRF5* gene encodes the type 5 regulation factor, a transcription factor involved in signaling by Toll-like receptors (TLRs) and in activation of type I interferon. A number of *IFR5* variants have been shown to be associated with SSc [8]. IL-1ß in SSc is also important.

TLRs are a class of proteins that play an important role in the innate immune system. They are single, membrane-spanning, non-catalytic receptors usually expressed in sentinel cells. TLR2 was associated with anti-topoisomerase positivity, the diffuse cutaneous subtype of the disease and with the development of pulmonary arterial hypertention [9].

Several genetic studies have identified associations between variants of the *STAT4* gene and autoimmune diseases and this has been demonstrated in SSc [7]. *STAT4* expresses strong profibrotic effects by controlling T cell activation, proliferation and cytokine release.

Vascular Disorders

Raynaud phenomenon is a key element in vascular disorders.

Pulmonary arterial hypertension (PAH) is the main pulmonary vascular complication in patients with SSc, occurring in about 10% of cases, and is associated with increased mortality.

Many genes play a role in vascular tone, remodeling or angiogenesis, such as nitric oxide synthases, endothelin and its receptors, serotonin, angiotensin-converting enzyme or vascular endothelial growth factor.

Etiology

Exposure to silica dust, vinyl chloride, trichloroethylene, benzene, xylene, toluene are environmental factors, that play a very important role.

Microchimerism is the presence of a small number of circulating cells transferred from one individual to another during pregnancy, blood transfusion, blood-marrow and solid organs transplants. These cells may become activated by the second event, producing a graft versus-host reaction, which may trigger SSc.

Infectious agents such as cytomegalovirus, herpes viruses and retroviruses may be triggering factors.

Oxidative stress with associated generation of free radicals may also contribute to the etiology.

Pathogenesis

In the pathogenesis of SSc three main mechanisms are important:

1- Vascular damage, mainly in microcirculation, 2 - Immune system activation/inflammation and 3 - Fibrosis.

Vascular Damage Endothelial injury is caused by transforming growth factor beta (TGFβ) cytokine and intercellular adhesion molecule 1 (ICAM 1), produced by activated lymphocytes and endothelial cells (AECA).

Endothelial damage causes loss of normal vasomotor tone regulation (vasodilators decrease *e.g.* nitric oxide and vasoconstrictors increase, *e.g.* endothelin), inflammatory cell chemoattraction and adhesion. Exposure of sub-endothelial cells to RBC's results in fibrin deposition and intravascular thrombus formation.

Vasculopathy consists of fibrointimal proliferation of small vessels and vasospastic episodes triggered by cold or stress, which can lead to tissue ischemia.

Immune Activation/Inflammation

Autoimmune dysregulation includes lymphocyte activation that produces autoantibody, cytokine and chemokine release, and dysregulation of the innate immune system.

The presence of **ANA** can be found in more than 90% of patients with SSc. **Anti-Scl-70 antibodies** react with nuclear enzyme DNA topoisimerase I and are found in 30-40% of patients with **dcSSc. Anticentromere antibodies** (ACA) are present in 80-90% of patients with **lcSSc** and recognize protein components of the three-laminar kinetochore. Anti-RNA polymerases II and III are less common and found in patients with rapidly progressive disease and severe internal organ involvement.

Fibrosis is the final mechanism of SSc. It is due to an increased fibroblast production of collagen, especially types 1 and 3. The constant activation of collagen genes differentiate the uncontrolled fibrosis of SSc from normal response to injury. TGFβ plays an important role in the development of fibrosis. Fibrosis result in internal organ dysfunction.

The systemic manifestations are different, but the disease starts with Raynaud's phenomenon. In lcSSc Raynaud's phenomenon appears before the onset of disease by several years, but in diffuse pattern of scleroderma, the onset of scleroderma takes place after the first episode of Raynaud's phenomenon.

Patients may have overlapping symptoms, where scleroderma is accompanied by other autoimmune diseases such as systemic lupus erythematosus, polymyositis, Sjogren's syndrome or autoimmune thyroid disease.

CLINICAL MANIFESTATIONS

General Manifestations

Fatigue, malaise, arthralgias and myalgias are common symptoms in SSc.

Skin Manifestations

The earliest sign of skin involvement is Raynaud's phenomenon.

Puffy hands are another sign, which is characterized by swelling of the fingers. The oedema is caused by increased vascular permeability. Finger mobility is restricted [10]. Puffy hands resemble oedema due to congestive heart failure or obstruction of veins.

Sclerodactyly is a sign with restricted mobility.

"Hard skin" due to fibrosis or sclerosis is seen. This is due to the loss of cutaneous elasticity and tightness, making the skin hard.

Sclerosis develops gradually and starts with oedema and later develops into sclerosis, resulting in atrophy.

Fibrosis involves all structures in the skin, including vessels and skin appendages (hair follicles, sweat glands) and leads to their narrowing or atrophy and eventually loss. The skin appears stretched and shiny and the skin's color may also change.

Facial features include teleangiectasies, a beak-shaped nose, reduced oral orifice of the mouth (microistomy) and radial furrowing around the mouth. Sclerosis also includes the lips. Fibrosis results in hardening of the face so that the patient has difficulty showing facial expressions and emotion resulting in a mask-like face.

Skin involvement is assess by skin thickness, pliability and fixation. The modified Rodman skin score is used to grade the severity of these features from 0 (normal) to 3 (severe) in 17 different areas of the body: face, anterior chest, abdomen, (right and left separatery) fingers, forearms, upper arms, tights, lower legs, dorsum of hands and feet. These individual values are added and the sum is definied as the total skin score [11].

Other skin manifestations include:

Scleroedema in the early stage

Pruritus in the early stage

Teleangiectasia, especially on the face

Digital ulcers

Pitting at the fingertips

Calcinosis cutis

Depigmentation and hyperpigmentation.

Limited cutaneous SSc is restricted to the face, neck and area distal to the elbows and knees.

Diffuse cutaneous SSc is distribution of sclerotic skin affecting other areas in addition to those affected by limited disease.

Systemic organ fibrosis may cause reduced function, which may lead to end-stage organ failure.

Differential Diagnosis of Scleroderma

Scleroderma-like skin changes may occur in the following conditions:

1. Localised scleroderma (morphea) and its variants (eosinophilic fasciitis - sudden onset of sclerosis involving the subculaneous tissue mainly in the extremities, peripheral eosinophilia); they do not include signs of systemic involvement or Raynaud's phenomenon.
2. Scleromyxedema in patients with dysfunction of the thyroid.
3. Scleroderma adultorum Buschke leads to non-pitting scleroedema. The skin

cannot be indented by pressure of the fingers; it occurs in patients with uncontrolled diabetes mellitus.
4. Nephrogenic systemic fibrosis is a scleroderma-like syndrome which occurs in patients with renal insufficiency who have received gadolinium based contrast.
5. Scleroderma-like graft-versus-host disease.
6. Fibrosis of hands in porphyria cutanea tarda.
7. Fibrosis in toxic oil syndrome, after exposure to polyvinyl chloride or to organic solvents.

Raynaud's phenomenon (RP) is observed in 90-98% of SSc patients before the development of the disease. RP of the fingers, toes, ears, and nose is characterized by episodic attacks that cause the blood vessels in the fingers and toes to constrict. RP presents with three changes in skin color. Pallor is a response to spasm of arterioles, next cyanosis is a result of ischemia and ending as a reperfusion dilation rub. Duration of an attack may last from less than one minute to several hours.

Nail fold capillary microscopy shows enlarged capillaries, bushy capillary formations, microhemorrhages and in the later stages loss of capillaries with or without avascular areas.

Fingertip ulceration is a complication of RP and occurs in 45% of patients with SSc. They heal slowly and become infected easily, leading to gangrene. As they deepen into the tissues, bone involvement may give osteomyelitis. Digital amputation may be required.

Gastrointestinal tract involvement The development of gastro-oesophageal reflux is an important problem due to the decreased pressure of the lower oesophageal sphincter Neutralisation of the gastric acid by saliva is decreased.

Symptoms of acid reflux requires endoscopy to identify strictures, stenosies, bacterial and fungal infection, Barrett's oesophagus and adenocarcinoma. Fibrosis involves the entire gastrointestinal tract and results in muscle wall atrophy. Damage to the gut's nervous system causes dysmotility and occurs in up to 90% of SSc patients. Stomach, small bowel, colon and anorectal involvement are present in 50% of SSc patients. Oesophageal involvement results in poor functioning of the muscle of the lower part of the oesophagus, reduction of peristalsis and laxity in the lower oesophageal sphincter. Symptoms include dysphagia, reflux, heartburn, pyrosis, and regurgitation. Barrett's oesophagus may occur. Oesophageal motility is tested by manometry. Small intestinal bacterial overgrowth syndrome is due to low colonization of bacteria in the upper GI tract that increases significantly. Bacterial transformation of nutrients into non-absorbable and toxic metabolites leads to malabsorption of fats, proteins, carbohydrates and vitamins and damage to the intestinal mucosa. Xylose breath test is used to detect these changes.

The stomach is less problematic in SSc but symptoms such as bloating, nausea, abdominal pain, diarrhea, fatty stool and anorexia have been observed. These are also based on gastric dysfunction and a reduction in gastric and antroduodenal emptying. Surface multi-channel electrogastrography has shown abnormalities of gastric myoelectric activity in patients with SSc, and correlations between electrogastrography and gastric emptying were also observed. Watermelon stomach is due to numerous ecstatic mucosal vessels leading to persistent blood loss and chronic anaemia and is characterized by multiple longitudinal lines of vessels, in the gastric antrum radiating from the pylorus to the antrum and through the stomach. Patients may show reduced emptying of the gall bladder, which decreases the pancreatobiliary function, and increases malabsorption, malnutrition and symptoms of the intestine and lower GIT. Faecal incontinence in SSc is frequent and is related to neuropathy. This is due to the absence of rectoanal inhibitory reflex assessment and higher anal sensory threshold. Primary biliary cirrhosis can occur in combination with limited SSc, and is called Reynold's syndrome.

Lung involvement The most important cause of morbidity and mortality in SSc patients is pulmonary involvement. The main types of lung involvement are alveolitis, membrane thickening and changes in microcirculation leading to interstitial lung disease (ILD) and pulmonary arterial hypertension (PAH). The symptoms of **pulmonary fibrosis** are dyspnea on exertion, non productive cough, hypoxemia, and haemoptysis. Breathlessness and dry cough are symptoms of SSc- ILD [12]. Breathlessness may be limited to exertion or present at rest, depending on the severity of lung disease. Non-productive cough is present in 30% of patient with SSc-ILD. Fine bibasilar crackles on chest auscultation are characteristic. The pulmonary function test (PFT) in SSc shows a restrictive pattern with a decreased forced vital capacity (FVC) or total lung capacity in spirometry. Pulmonary **carbon monoxide diffusion capacity (DLCO)** is reduced.

Bronchoalveolar lavage. Cytological analysis of bronchoalveolar lavage fluid (BALF) in SSc-ILD shows increased percentages of neutrophils, eosinophils and/or lymphocytes, and is also called alveolitis [13]. Chest high-resolution CT (HRCT) is a gold standard technique used for the diagnosis. Early changes of lung fibrosis are "ground glass", which is followed by "honeycombing" in cases of extensive fibrosis. HRCT may help in differential diagnosis of other conditions such as emphysema, reveal features of heart disease and may rule out or confirm pulmonary thromboembolism if used with contrast.

PAH is a life-threatening condition that can develop in patients with SSc. It occurs when the blood vessels supplying the lungs constrict and become stiffer and thicker due to irreversible fibrosis. The increased resistance in pulmonary circulation makes it difficult for blood to flow through to the lung vessels, and thus the heart must pump harder, leading to heart failure. PAH is a late complication of the lsSSc but occurs earlier in the dsSSc. The most common symptom of PAH is gradually progressive shortness of breath when patients exert themselves. Fatigue and weakness are common. Ankle swelling, nausea and abdominal swelling reflect right-sided heart failure. The early stages of PAH are asymptomatic. The first physical signs include a loud P2 which may be palpable. As the PAP and PVR increase, a pressure load is put on the right ventricle (RV), resulting in heart failure, tachycardia, cyanosis, raised venous pressure, murmur of tricuspid regurgitation, RV third sound, and an enlarged liver with oedema. Crepitations may indicate the presence of ILD. Dyspnea occurs with chest pain and syncope. Physical examination shows an increased second heart sound, a pansystolic murmur of tricuspid regurgitation, a diastolic murmur of pulmonary insufficiency and a right ventricular third sound. Doppler echocardiography should be performed annually, because asymptomatic patients with SSc should be diagnose with PAH. If PAH is suspected, right-heart catheterization must be performed and is confirmed when the blood pressure is higher than 25 mmHg in the pulmonary artery at rest. To assess exercise capacity in PAH patients, **6-minute walking test (6MWT)** is used. This test is simple, inexpensive and evaluates the distance walked, dyspnoea on exertion (Borg scale) and finger O_2 saturation. Walking distances <332 m and O_2 desaturation >10% indicates worse prognosis in PAH patients. Patients with PAH diagnosis live on average 2.8 years. **NT-pro BNP** is a biochemical marker used to monitor progress and/or response to treatment in patients with PAH.

Cardiac involvement is common in SSc but is often silent and involves both the myocardium and the conducting system. Primary heart disease is due to abnormal vasoreactivity in microcirculation. Symptoms are shortness of breath, chest pain, fatigue, and palpitations. Tachyarrhythmias are accompanied by irregular heart beats due to over-expression of the adrenergic system and renine-angiotensi--aldosterone system. Patients should undergo CV risk factors assessment, standard 12-lead ECG, 24 h Holter monitoring, Doppler echocardiography, tissue Doppler echocardiography, natriuretic peptides, and sometimes invasive electrophysiology studies, coronary angiography and right heart catheterization.

Myocardial involvement in scleroderma is detected by a single photon emission computed tomography (SPECT), radionuclide ventriculography, tissue Doppler echocardiography (TDE) and magnetic resonance imaging (MRI) [14]. Coronary atherosclerosis is similar to the general population [15]. Patients with SSc and normal coronary arteries may have angina pectoris and myocardial infarction due to impaired myocardial microcirculation. Repeated ischaemia-reperfusion abnormalities may lead to irreversible myocardial fibrosis [14]. Non-invasive transthoracic Doppler imaging before and after adenosine infusion have confirmed the presence of an impaired coronary flow reserve in SSc patients [16]. Vasospasm of the small coronary arteries or arterioles play a role in myocardial abnormalities in patients with SSc [14]. Vasospasm is reversible after intravenous administration of dipyridamole, and after treatment with nifedipine, nicardipine or captopril. Improved myocardial perfusion was seen using thalium-201 SPECT [14].

Fibrotic lesions, characteristic of late myocardial involvement in SSc, present in both ventricles and are not consistent with large coronary artery distribution [14]. Although advanced myocardial fibrosis may lead to congestive heart failure, systolic or diastolic dysfunction can occur early in the disease, many years before it becomes clinically evident. The long-term use of calcium channel blockers appeared to be protective against LV dysfunction in a large series of 7073 patients with SSc [17].

Pericarditis may be presented as asymptomatic pericardial effusion, revealed by echocardiography on routine examination, to severe fluid accumulation resulting in heart failure [18]. Most cases of pericardial changes are due to a SSc process, but also to uraemia in end-stage SSc [19]. Pericarditis is a bad prognostic factor with risk of death [20].

Renal manifestations of SSc. The most important manifestation is scleroderma renal crisis (SRC). In the past it was a common cause of SSc-related death. This complication is now treatable by ACE inhibitors [21].

Increased interstitial fibrillar collagen is present in SSc renal tissue. Half of patients of SSc may show a reduced glomerular filtration rate compared to age-matched healthy controls. Microscopic proteinuria both glomerular and trubular has been shown. Renal manifestations of SSc are interstitial nephritis, drug-related and glomerulonaphritis. Glomerulonephritis is seen in cases where there is serological evidence of overlap with systemic lupus erythematosus (SLE) or when there is a positive antineutrophil cytoplasmic antibody (ANCA) test [22]. The presence of ANCA in SSc should raise suspicion of inflammatory renal disease or vasculitis and a renal biopsy should be performed.

Scleroderma renal crisis (SRC) is defined as new onset of sudden arterial hypertension and/or rapidly progressive oliguric renal failure during the course of SSc. This life threatening complication develops in stable patients who suddenly develop severe arterial hypertension with headache, visual disturbance, seizures, signs of congestive heart failure, pericardial effusion, haemolytic anemia, thrombocytopenia and acute oliguric renal failure with microscopic hematuria. The optic fundus show acute hypertensive changes, such as haemorrhages and exudates in the optic fundi.

Sometimes SRC symptoms may be non-specific – a patient may report increased fatigue, headache, dyspnoea or just a general feeling of being unwell. Patients at high risk must be taught to take these symptoms seriously and should check their own blood pressure at the onset of SRC.

Joint Involvement In some patients joint synovitis, joint contracture and tendon friction rubs have been observed. Manifestations ranging from arthralgia to arthritis, contactures and tendon friction rubs. Articular involvement contributes to disability and impaired quality of life in SSc, reducing ability to work or perform activities of daily living [23]. Osteoarticular, muscle and soft tissue involvement may impair hand function secondary to stiff/painful joints and reduced dexterity and/or grip [24].

Symptoms of joint involvement can precedes the onset of Raynaud's phenomenon or occur concurrently with it, and therefore may be an early indicator of SSc. It is very important to note that patients presenting only with articular involvement (arthralgia, synovitis or tenosynovitis), to look for early signs of SSc, such as Raynaud's phenomenon and puffy fingers.

Generalised arthralgia with slight pain and stiffness are the most frequent articular symptoms of SSc. In very early diffuse cutaneous SSc, arthralgia may be difficult to evaluate because of rapidly progressing skin involvement leading to skin tightening and pain.

Onset may be acute or chronic with one or more joint involvement. Most joints can be involved, with the fingers (in particular the metacarpophalangeal (MCP) and the proximal interphalangeal (PIP) joints), wrists and ankles predominantly affected. As the cutaneous involvement progresses, there is tightening and a contracture of the underlying joints with impairment of movement and function. Joint contracture, resulting from joint destruction may evolve into ankylosis and fibrotic changes in the skin. Some patients show localized joint tenderness or swelling, and joint effusions.

Up to 30% of SSc patients are positive for rheumatoid factor [25]. Testing for anti-cyclic citrullinated peptide (anti-CCP) antibodies might be of great help in identifying the infrequent cases of true SSc-rheumatoid arthritis overlap [26]. Synovitis may be a predictive factor for the diffuse cutaneous subset and poor prognosis [27].

Radiographic abnormalities have been seen in patients with SSc. Articular lesions, juxta-articular osteoporosis, joint space narrowing and erosions, have been observed in the MCP, PIP and distal interphalangeal (DIP) joints, as well as the wrist. SSc arthropathy may present as those resembling erosive osteoarthritis or psoriatic arthritis with relative sparing of MCP joints to that of changes similar to RA.

Pensil-in-cup deformity in hands and feet may be associated with non-articular abnormalities, such as skin atrophy, subcutaneous calcinosis and digital tuft resorption [25].

Tendon abnormalities are described as "leathery crepitus" on palpation of the knees, wrists, fingers and ankles during motion. In the lower extremities, tendon rubs are usually localized to the tendons of the tibialis anterior and the Achilles tendon or the peronaeus muscles. In the forearm, the source of the rub is due to tendons of the flexor or extensor muscles immediately proximal to the wrist. Tendon involvement is more prevalent in patients with diffuse cutaneous form of SSc and early disease [26].

Subcutaneous calcifications are a hallmark of SSc. Calcinosis may also occur in feet, knees and legs. There is a link between calcinosis, acro-osteolysis and digital ulcerations. Myopathy is common in SSc, affecting up to 80% of SSc patients.

TREATMENT

Severe forms of the disease and rapidly progressive diffuse SSc with pulmonary, cardiac, and renal involvement, are associated with a high mortality rate, estimated at 40-50% in 5 years. There is no proven effective treatment to stop fibrosis and disease progression beside autologous haemopoietic stem cell transplantation (AHSCT). Cyclophospamide is the only drug considered to have moderate efficacy in patients with ILD. Treatment of specific organs is very important.

PAH is treated by the endothelin pathway using endothelin receptor blocking agents with the nitric oxide pathway using phosphodiesterase-5 inhibitors and the prostacyclin pathway using prostanoids.

Using combination therapy with all three pathways is necessary in patients because PAH is a progressive condition and patients deteriorate despite therapy.

In **PAH** vasoreactive agents like calcium channel blockers (nifedipine, diltiazem), non-vasoreactive agents, such as endothelin receptor antagonists – bosentan, sitaxentan, ambrisentan, followed by PDE5 inhibitor – sildenafil (Viagra) or tadalafil and prostaglandins iv prostacyclin (epoprostenol, PGI2), sc, inhaled (ex. inhaled-solution form of iloprost or treprostinil) are used. Anticoagulation, usually warfarin, is recommended for most patients with PAH because prothrombotic coagulation abnormalities, abnormalities in the fibrinolytic and coagulation pathways, endothelial abnormalities, and the general prothrombotic factors such as immobility and heart failure is observed.

International normalized ratio (INR) levels are kept between 2 and 3 in the USA and UK and 1,5 to 2.5 in Europe.

Diuretics – Symptomatic relief is observed in patients with fluid overload.

Oxygen therapy reduces dyspnoea and improves exercise capacity in patients with severe hypoxia.

In **pericarditis** immobilisation and non-steroidal anti-inflammatory drug treatment (indometacin 25 – 50 mg orally, aspirin 300- 650 mg every 4 – 6 h or ibuprofen 600 – 800 mg three times daily) relieve the symptoms. However, in patients with severe pain or symptoms persisting for longer than 48 h administration of steroids (prednisone 60 – 80 mg, tapering to zero over 1 week) may be necessary. Colchicine (1.2 mg twice a day, or 1 mg daily after a 2 – 3 mg loading dose) may be added to taper patients off corticosteroids.

In cases of tamponade, needle puncture and drainage of the effusion are performed. Surgical pericardial window may be necessary when pericardial effusion occurs repeatedly [18].

In **gastro-intestinal involvement** modifications in lifestyle, (*e.g.* upright posture maintained until a meal is digested), and diet with reduced fats and fibers is very important. Oesophageal dysmotility and reflux are treated with promotility agents, H2 blockers, and proton pump inhibitors (*e.g.* omeprazol). In bacterial overgrowth syndrome broad-spectrum antibiotics such us ciprofloxacin, metronidazol, cephalosporins must be used for a few days each month. The lack of prokinetic ability requires the use of prokinetics and acid blockers.

In **digital vasculopathy** patients must avoid smoking, beta-blockers, cold and stress. Some improvement is observed after using nifedipine, iloprost, bosentan.

Kidney involvement Patients who develop high blood pressure should immediately receive ACE inhibitors. Patients who lose renal function need dialysis.

Prophylactic use of ACE inhibitors and daily at-home monitoring of blood pressure is suggested to prevent sudden kidney failure. Regular assessment of urine and biochemical markers of renal function is important. New-onset hypertension in patients with SSc should be treated with ACE inhibitors.

Arthralgia is treated with non-steroidal anti-inflammatory drug (NSAID). Low dose corticosteroids (<10 mg/day) may be used for the symptomatic treatment of inflammatory arthritis or tenosynovitis, although there is a risk of renal crisis. Methotrexate may be used for the treatment of inflammatory arthritis.

The treatment of **tendon involvement** is usually symptomatic and supportive. Tenosinovitis will respond to NSAIDs or low doses of corticosteroids.

Autologous haemopoietic stem cell transplantation (AHSCT) following bone marrow ablation has been used to treat serious cases.

EULAR recommendations for the treatment of systemic sclerosis: a report from the EULAR Scleroderma Trials and Research group (EUSTAR) [28]

Recommendation

I. SSc-related digital vasculopathy (Raynaud's phenomenon [RP], digital ulcers):

1. A meta-analysis on dihydropirine-type calcium antagonists and one meta-analysis on prostanoids indicate that nifedipine and intravenous iloprost reduce the frequency and severity of SSc-RP attacks Dihydropiridine-type calcium antagonists, usually oral nifedipine, should be considered for first-line therapy for SSc-RP, and intravenous iloprost, or other available intravenous prostanoids for severe SSc-RP.

2. Two RCT indicate that intravenous prostanoids (particularly intravenous iloprost) are efficacious in healing digital ulcers in patients with SSc. Intravenous prostanoids (in particular iloprost) should be considered in the treatment of active digital ulcers in patients with SSc.

3. Bosentan has no confirmed efficacy in the treatment of active digital ulcers in SSc patients. Bosentan has confirmed efficacy in two high-quality randomized controlled trial (RCT) to prevent digital ulcers in diffuse SSc patients, in particular in those with multiple digital ulcers.

Bosentan should be considered in diffuse SSc with multiple digital ulcers after failure of calcium antagonists and, usually, prostanoid therapy.

II. SSc- PAH (SSc-related pulmonary arterial hypertension):

4. Two high-quality RCT indicated that bosentan improves exercise capacity,

functional class and some haemodynamic measures in PAH. At present Bosentan should be strongly considered to treat SSc-PAH.

5. Two high-quality RCT indicated that sitaxentan improves exercise capacity, functional class and some haemodynamic measures in PAH. At present, sitaxentan may also be considered to treat SSc-PAH.

6. One high-quality RCT indicates that sildenafil improves exercise capacity, functional class and some haemodynamic measure in PAH. Sildenafil may be considered to treat SSc-PAH.

7. One high-quality RCT indicates that continous intravenous epoprostenol improves exercise capacity, functional class and haemodynamic measure in SSc-PAH. Sudden drug withdrawal may be life threatening.

Intravenous epoprostenol should be considered to treatment of patients with severe SSc-PAH.

III. SSc-related skin involvement:

8. Two RCT have shown that methotrexate improves skin score in early diffuse SSc. Positive effects on other organ manifestations have not been established.

Methotrexate may be considered for treatment of skin manifestations of early diffuse SSc.

IV. SSc-ILD (SSc-related interstitial lung disease):

9. In view of the results from two high-quality RCT and despite its known toxicity, cyclophosphamide should be considered for treatment of SSc-ILD.

V. Scleroderma renal crisis:

10. Despite the lack of RCT, expert believe that ACE inhibitors should be used in the treatment of SRC.

11. Four retrospective studies suggest that steroids are associated with a higher risk of SRC. Patients on steroids should be carefully monitored for blood pressure and renal function.

VI. SSc-related gastrointestinal disease:

12. Despite the lack of specific RCT, experts believe that PPI should be used for the prevention of SSc-related gastrooesophageal reflux, oesophageal ulcers and strictures.

13. Despite the lack of specific RCT, experts believe that prokinetic drugs should be used for the management of SSc-related symptomatic motility disturbances (dysphagia, gastro-oesophageal reflux disease [GORD], early satiety, bloating, pseudo-obstruction, *etc.*).

14. Despite the lack of specific RCT, experts believe that, when malabsorption is caused by bacterial overgrowth, rotating antibiotics may be useful in SSc patients.

REFERENCES

[1]   Masi AT, Rodnan GP, Medsger TA, *et al.* Preliminary criteria for the classification of systemic sclerosis (scleroderma). Subcommittee for scleroderma criteria of the American Rheumatism Association Diagnostic and Therapeutic Criteria Committee. Arthritis Rheum 1980; 23(5): 581-90.
[http://dx.doi.org/10.1002/art.1780230510] [PMID: 7378088]

[2]   van den Hoogen F, Khanna D, Fransen J, *et al.* 2013 classification criteria for systemic sclerosis: an American College of Rheumatology/European League against Rheumatism collaborative initiative. Arthritis Rheum 2013; 65(11): 2737-47.
[http://dx.doi.org/10.1002/art.38098] [PMID: 24122180]

[3]   Vonk MC, Broers B, Heijdra YF, *et al.* Systemic sclerosis and its pulmonary complications in The Netherlands: an epidemiological study. Ann Rheum Dis 2009; 68(6): 961-5.
[http://dx.doi.org/10.1136/ard.2008.091710] [PMID: 18511546]

[4]   Silman AJ. Scleroderma-demographics and survival. J Rheumatol Suppl 1997; 48: 58-61.
[PMID: 9150120]

[5]   Arnett FC, Cho M, Chatterjee S, Aguilar MB, Reveille JD, Mayes MD. Familial occurrence frequencies and relative risks for systemic sclerosis (scleroderma) in three United States cohorts. Arthritis Rheum 2001; 44(6): 1359-62.
[http://dx.doi.org/10.1002/1529-0131(200106)44:6<1359::AID-ART228>3.0.CO;2-S]   [PMID: 11407695]

[6]   Manetti M, Guiducci S, Ibba-Manneschi L, Matucci-Cerinic M. Mechanisms in the loss of capillaries in systemic sclerosis: angiogenesis versus vasculogenesis. J Cell Mol Med 2010; 14(6A): 1241-54.
[http://dx.doi.org/10.1111/j.1582-4934.2010.01027.x] [PMID: 20132409]

[7]   Radstake TR, Gorlova O, Rueda B, *et al.* Genome-wide association study of systemic sclerosis identifies CD247 as a new susceptibility locus. Nat Genet 2010; 42(5): 426-9.
[http://dx.doi.org/10.1038/ng.565] [PMID: 20383147]

[8]   Dieudé P, Guedj M, Wipff J, *et al.* Association between the IRF5 rs2004640 functional polymorphism and systemic sclerosis: a new perspective for pulmonary fibrosis. Arthritis Rheum 2009; 60(1): 225-33.
[http://dx.doi.org/10.1002/art.24183] [PMID: 19116937]

[9]   Broen JC, Bossini-Castillo L, van Bon L, *et al.* A rare polymorphism in the gene for Toll-like receptor 2 is associated with systemic sclerosis phenotype and increases the production of inflammatory mediators. Arthritis Rheum 2012; 64(1): 264-71.
[http://dx.doi.org/10.1002/art.33325] [PMID: 21905008]

[10]   Avouac J, Fransen J, Walker UA, *et al.* Preliminary criteria for the very early diagnosis of systemic sclerosis: results of a Delphi Consensus Study from EULAR Scleroderma Trials and Research Group. Ann Rheum Dis 2011; 70(3): 476-81.
[http://dx.doi.org/10.1136/ard.2010.136929] [PMID: 21081523]

[11]   Clements PJ, Lachenbruch PA, Seibold JR, *et al.* Skin thickness score in systemic sclerosis: an assessment of interobserver variability in 3 independent studies. J Rheumatol 1993; 20(11): 1892-6.
[PMID: 8308774]

[12]   Bussone G, Mouthon L. Interstitial lung disease in systemic sclerosis. Autoimmun Rev 2011; 10(5): 248-55.
[http://dx.doi.org/10.1016/j.autrev.2010.09.012] [PMID: 20863911]

[13]   Wells AU. The clinical utility of bronchoalveolar lavage in diffuse parenchymal lung disease. Eur Respir Rev 2010; 19(117): 237-41.
[http://dx.doi.org/10.1183/09059180.00005510] [PMID: 20956199]

[14]   Meune C, Vignaux O, Kahan A, Allanore Y. Heart involvement in systemic sclerosis: evolving concept and diagnostic methodologies. Arch Cardiovasc Dis 2010; 103(1): 46-52.
[http://dx.doi.org/10.1016/j.acvd.2009.06.009] [PMID: 20142120]

[15]   Au K, Singh MK, Bodukam V, *et al.* Atherosclerosis in systemic sclerosis: a systematic review and meta-analysis. Arthritis Rheum 2011; 63(7): 2078-90.
[http://dx.doi.org/10.1002/art.30380] [PMID: 21480189]

[16]   Montisci R, Vacca A, Garau P, *et al.* Detection of early impairment of coronary flow reserve in patients with systemic sclerosis. Ann Rheum Dis 2003; 62(9): 890-3.
[http://dx.doi.org/10.1136/ard.62.9.890] [PMID: 12922965]

[17]   Allanore Y, Meune C, Vonk MC, *et al.* Prevalence and factors associated with left ventricular dysfunction in the EULAR Scleroderma Trial and Research group (EUSTAR) database of systemic sclerosis patients. Ann Rheum Dis 2010; 69: 218-21.
[http://dx.doi.org/10.1136/ard.2008.103382] [PMID: 19279015]

[18]   Nabatian S, Kantola R, Sabri N, Broy S, Lakier JB. Recurrent pericardial effusion and pericardial tamponade in a patient with limited systemic sclerosis. Rheumatol Int 2007; 27(8): 759-61.
[http://dx.doi.org/10.1007/s00296-006-0277-2] [PMID: 17351776]

[19]   Biholong AE, Allagui E, Delforge ML, Vandergheynst F, Renard M. [Acute pericarditis in a sclerodermic patient at the 27th week of pregnancy]. Rev Med Brux 2009; 30(6): 588-91.
[PMID: 20545072]

[20]   Martini G, Vittadello F, Kasapçopur O, *et al.* Factors affecting survival in juvenile systemic sclerosis. Rheumatology (Oxford) 2009; 48(2): 119-22.
[http://dx.doi.org/10.1093/rheumatology/ken388] [PMID: 18854345]

[21]   Steen VD, Syzd A, Johnson JP, Greenberg A, Medsger TA Jr. Kidney disease other than renal crisis in patients with diffuse scleroderma. J Rheumatol 2005; 32(4): 649-55.
[PMID: 15801020]

[22]   Arnaud L, Huart A, Plaisier E, *et al.* ANCA-related crescentic glomerulonephritis in systemic sclerosis: revisiting the "normotensive scleroderma renal crisis". Clin Nephrol 2007; 68(3): 165-70.
[http://dx.doi.org/10.5414/CNP68165] [PMID: 17915619]

[23]   Mau W, Listing J, Huscher D, Zeidler H, Zink A. Employment across chronic inflammatory rheumatic diseases and comparison with the general population. J Rheumatol 2005; 32(4): 721-8.
[PMID: 15801031]

[24]   Sandqvist G, Eklund M, Akesson A, Nordenskiöld U. Daily activities and hand function in women with scleroderma. Scand J Rheumatol 2004; 33(2): 102-7.
[http://dx.doi.org/10.1080/03009740410006060] [PMID: 15163111]

[25]   Avouac J, Guerini H, Wipff J, *et al.* Radiological hand involvement in systemic sclerosis. Ann Rheum Dis 2006; 65(8): 1088-92.
[http://dx.doi.org/10.1136/ard.2005.044602] [PMID: 16414976]

[26]   Avouac J, Gossec L, Dougados M. Diagnostic and predictive value of anti-cyclic citrullinated protein antibodies in rheumatoid arthritis: a systematic literature review. Ann Rheum Dis 2006; 65(7): 845-51.
[http://dx.doi.org/10.1136/ard.2006.051391] [PMID: 16606649]

[27]   Avouac J, Walker U, Tyndall A, *et al.* Characteristics of joint involvement and relationships with

systemic inflammation in systemic sclerosis: results from the EULAR Scleroderma Trial and Research Group (EUSTAR) database. J Rheumatol 2010; 37(7): 1488-501.
[http://dx.doi.org/10.3899/jrheum.091165] [PMID: 20551097]

[28]   Kowal-Bielecka O, Fransen J, Avouac J, *et al.* Update of EULAR recommendations for the treatment of systemic sclerosis. Ann Rheum Dis 2017; 76(8): 1327-39.
[http://dx.doi.org/10.1136/annrheumdis-2016-209909] [PMID: 27941129]

CHAPTER 8

Vasculitis

Abstract: Vasculitis is inflammation in vessel walls leading to poor blood circulation and damage to vessels. The vasculitis are devided into large vessel vasculitis (Takayasu arteritis [TAK] and Giant cell arteritis [GCA]), medium vessel vasculitis (Polyarteritis nodosa and Kawasaki disease), small vessel vasculitis associated with antineutrophil cytoplasmic antibody (microscopic polyangiitis [MPA], granulomatosis with polyangiitis [GPA], eosinophilic granulomatosis with polyangiitis [EGPA]) and others.

TAK affects patients younger than 50 years, and GCA after age 50. Clinical features include leg claudication, headaches, postural dizziness, visual disturbances and reduced or absent upper limb pulses.

Management of TAK and GCA include high doses of GCS. Treatment of GCA can prevent blindness due to occlusion of optic arteries. New option is tocilizumab.

Polyarteritis nodosa inflammation involves the skin, kidneys, peripheral nerves, muscles, and gut in patients between 40-60 years old. Management includes GCS, CYC and AZA.

Kawasaki disease is an acute febrile mucocutaneous and lymph node disease affecting young children. Coronary arteries are often involved. Management includes IVIG and aspirin.

GPA is necrotizing granulomatous inflammation involving the upper and lower respiratory tract, necrotizing glomerulonephritis, ocular vasculitis, pulmonary capillaritis with hemorrhage and granulomatous and nongranulomatous extravascular inflammation is common. c-ANCA is present in 98% of patients. Management is high doses of GCS, CYC, rituximab and AZA.

EGPA is characterized by pulmonary and systemic small vessel vasculitis, granulomas and hypereosinophilia. Clinical features are atopic history, asthma, allergic rhinitis, pulmonary infiltrates, mono/polyneuropathy, mononeuritis multiplex, purpura and eosinophilia. Management is high doses of GCS, CYC and AZA.

Keywords: Antineutrophil cytoplasmic antibody, AZA, CYC, Eosinophilic granulomatosis with polyangiitis [EGPA], GCS, Giant cell arteritis [GCA], Granulomatosis with polyangiitis [GPA], Kawasaki disease, Large vessel vasculitis, Medium vessel vasculitis, Microscopic polyangiitis [MPA], Polyarteritis nodosa, Rituximab, Small vessel vasculitis, Takayasu arteritis [TAK], Vasculitis.

INTRODUCTION

Vasculitis is inflammation in or through vessel walls leading to poor blood circulation and damage to the vessel integrity. Involvement includes one, or many organ systems. Destruction of the vessel wall in vasculitis is seen histologically as fibrinoid necrosis, hence the term "necrotizing vasculitis".

Symptoms are a result of ischaemia of tissue, fever, weight loss, anorexia and inflammation. It is important what kind of vessels are involved in the inflammatory process what is included in the last nomenclature of vasculitis.

Name for vasculitides adopted by the 2012 International Chapel Hill Consensus Conference on the Nomenclature of Vasculitides [1]:

Large vessel vasculitis (LVV)

Takayasu arteritis (TAK)

Giant cell arteritis (GCA)

Medium vessel vasculitis (MVV)

Polyarteritis nodosa (PAN)

Kawasaki disease (KD)

Small vessel vasculitis (SVV)

Antineutrophil cytoplasmic antibody (ANCA)– associated vasculitis (AAV)

Microscopic polyangiitis (MPA)

Granulomatosis with polyangiitis (GPA)

Eosinophilic granulomatosis with polyangiitis (EGPA).

Immune complex SVV

Anti-glomerular basement membrane (anti-GBM) disease

Cryoglobulinemic vasculitis (CV)

IgA vasculitis (IgAV)

Hypocomplementemic urticarial vasculitis(HUV)(anti-C1q vasculitis)

Variable vessel vasculitis (VVV)

Behcet's disease (BD)

Cogan's syndrome (CS)

Single-organ vasculitis (SOV)

Cutaneous leukocytoclastic angiitis

Cutaneous arteritis

Primary central nervous system vasculitis

Isolated aortitis

Others

Vasculitis associated with systemic disease

Lupus vasculitis

Rheumatoid vasculitis

Sarcoid vasculitis

Others

Vasculitis associated with probable etiology

Hepatitis C virus-associated cryoglobulinemic vasculitis

Hepatitis B virus-associated vasculitis

Syphilis-associated aortitis

Drug-associated immune complex vasculitis

Drug-associated ANCA-associated vasculitis

Cancer-associated vasculitis

Others

International Chapel Hill Consensus Conference on the Nomenclature of Vasculitides (CHCC2012) adopted the definition for vasculitides in 2012 [1].

LARGE VESSEL VASCULITIS (LVV)

Vasculitis affecting large arteries more common than other vasculitides. Large arteries include the aorta and its major branches.

Takayashu Arteritis (TAK) is a granulomatous vasculitis of unknown etiology, affecting the aorta, its major branches and the pulmonary arteries. It affects patients younger than 50 years, which differs from giant cell arteritis, whose onset occurs after age 50. It affects mostly women of Eastern ethnic background under 40 years of age, mainly between 15-25 years old, with sex ratio men to women = 1: 9.

At the time of diagnosis, approximately 20% of patients with TAK are clinically asymptomatic [2]. On physical examination, the most frequent features are bruits, diminished or absent pulses and asymmetrical blood pressure measurements between extremities. Hypertension has been reported and it is an important cause of morbidity in TAK and contributes to cardiac, cerebral and renal injury.

Clinical features are divided into systemic and occlusive phases. In the systemic phase patients have malaise, weight loss, fever, night sweats, fatigue, arthralgias and myalgias. In the occlusive phase there are arm or leg claudication, headaches, postural dizziness and visual disturbances. Reduced or absent upper limb pulses, decreased pulses and subclavian/aortic bruits.

Inflammation in vessels may lead to stenosis or formation of aneurysm. Symptoms of arterial stenosis include those of diminished blood flow to areas supplied by the vessel affected. Rupture, valvular incompetence may occur when the aortic root is involved. Decreased circulation to the extremities may present as intermittent claudication. Stenosis or occlusion of the carotids or vertebral arteries may decrease perfusion and cause injury to the brain and central nervous system. It may be asymptomatic or present with transient ischemic attacks, stroke, dizziness, syncope, headache or visual changes. Mesenteric involvement is common in TAK, and gastrointestinal symptoms such as nausea, diarrhea, vomiting and abdominal pain occur less frequently.

Cardiac involvement may present as dyspnea, palpitations, angina, myocardial infarction, heart failure and sudden death. Renal involvement is characterized by renovascular hypertension.

American College of Rheumatology classification criteria for Takayasu arteritis [3]:

CRITERION	DEFINITION
1. Age <40 years old	Development of symptoms or signs related to Takayasu arteritis at age <40 years
2. Claudication of extremities	Development and worsening of fatigue and discomfort in muscles of one or more extremities while in use, especially the upper extremities
3. Decreased brachial arterial pulse	Decreased pulsation of one or more extremity while in use, especially the upper extremities
4. Blood pressure difference > 10 mm Hg	Difference of > 10 mm Hg in systolic blood pressure between arms
5. Bruit over subclavian arteries or aorta	Bruit audible on auscultation over one or both subclavian arteries or abdominal aorta
6. Arteriogram abnormality	Arteriographic narrowing or occlusion of the entire aorta, its proximal branches, or large arteries in the proximal upper or lower extremities, not due to atherosclerosis, fibromuscular dysplasia or similar causes; changes usually focal or segmental.

Diagnosis of Takayashu arteritis requires at least three of six criteria to be present. The presence of any three or more criteria gives a sensitivity of 90,5% and specificity of 97,8% [3].

TAK is diagnosed by presence of arterial lesions in the aorta and its branches, that are characteristic and other causes of large vessel abnormalities have been excluded such as giant cell arteritis, Behcet's syndrome, Cogan's syndrome, Kawasaki's disease, sarcoidosis, rheumatoid arthritis, spondyloarthropathies, relapsing polychondritis, systemic lupus erythematosus, thromboangiitis obliterans infections, atherosclerosis, thromboembolism and others like as Ehlers-Danlos syndrome, Marfan's syndrome, neurofibromatosis, congenital aortic coarctation, fibromuscular dysplasia, radiation fibrosis, traumatic stenosis and ergotism.

Disease activity is assessed by evaluating imaging and clinical studies, symptoms, signs and laboratories. There is no laboratory study that is diagnostic for TAK or correlates with disease activity. The most common laboratory studies correlate with acute inflammation. The complete blood count may indicate a normochromic, normocytic anemia, leukocytosis and thrombocytosis.

Diagnostic imaging is important to diagnose TAK and is used for disease monitoring. Magnetic resonance angiography is used for assessing vessel patency in TAK. Arteriography using catheter-directed intravascular injection of contrast dye may show vascular luminar dimensions. Ultrasonography may show carotid lesions. Positron emission tomography (PET) may show cellular activity within an inflamed arterial wall.

Management includes high doses of GCS – prednisone 1 mg/kg/day (60 mg/daily) for the first 1-3 months, then over the next 2-3 months the dose is tapered and eventually discontinued. Methotrexate is used in a glucocorticoid-resistent patients in a maximum dose 25 mg once a week. Cyclophosphamide is used in patients who have active inflammatory disease in which glucocorticosteroids are effective but cannot be tapered and where the patient is unresponsive or intolerant to or unable to take MTX. Other immunosuppressive drugs include azathioprine, mycophenlate mofetil or leflunomide.

Surgery should be considered to revascularize stenosed or occluded vessels that cause ischemia. Indications for surgery include cerebral hypoperfusion, renovascular hypertention, limb claudicationm repair of aneurysms or valvular insufficiency. Now in TAK a new option for therapy is the IL-6R blocker tocilizumapb.

Giant Cell Arteritis (GCA) – Granulomatous arteritis affecting the aorta and/or its major branches, especially the branches of the carotid and vertebral arteries. The temporal artery is also often involved. The onset is usually in patients older than 50 years and is often associated with polymyalgia rheumatica. Giant cells are observed in biopsy specimens from patients with active GCA. The term "temporal arteritis" should not be used for patients with GCA because not all patients have temporal artery involvement, and other types of vasculitis can also affect the temporal arteries.

GCA occurs in patients between 60-75 years old, sex ratio men: women = 1: 3. Early recognition and treatment can prevent blindness and other complications due to occlusion or rupture of optic arteries. Features include fatigue, headaches, loss of vision, tongue or jaw claudication, hip or shoulder girdle stiffness, diplopia, scalp tenderness, polymyalgia rheumatica and aortic arch syndrome.

Headache is the most common symptom of the vasculitic process. It has a sudden onset, is severe and is located usually around the temporal area, but may affect any part of the head like as occipital, frontal and parietal regions. Pain is usually continuous, particularly at night, and sometimes responds to painkillers. Scalp tenderness occurs in around a third to a half of patients and is noticed while brushing or combing the hair. Physical examination in GCA may show tenderness, thickening, and nodules of the superficial temporal arteries. Temporal artery pulses may be decreased or absent. Sometimes bruits may be heard in the supra-aortic branches.

GCA is a major cause of irreversible visual loss. The most common ophthalmic manifestation of GCA is anterior ischemic optic neuropathy (AION). This is caused by interruption of blood flow in the posterior ciliary arteries to the optic nerve head. It is sudden painless loss of vision. Visual loss may present as a mist in the entire field or part of the visual field and evolve within 24-48 h to complete blindness. One eye is affected first, but involvement of the other eye in untreated patients may occur 1-10 days after the initial event. In the acute phase of AION, the optic disc is pale and swollen but the retina is almost normal. Rarely, visual loss is caused by central retinal artery occlusion, ischemic retrobulbar neuropathy or occipital infarction in association with a stroke involving the vertebrobasilar area.

Thoracic aorta aneurysms, abdominal aorta aneurysms and large vessel stenoses are found in patients with GCA. Aortic murmurs and vascular bruits in the arms, upper extremity claudication, hypertension, hyperlipidaemia, PMR and coronary artery disease are observed. Neuropathies such as mononeuropathies and peripheral polyneuropathies of the upper or lower extremities may also occur. Transient ischemic attacks and strokes caused by severe occlusion of the internal carotid artery or the vertebral arteries have been reported [4].

American College of Rheumatology classification criteria for giant-cell arteritis [5]:

CRITERION	DEFINITION
1. Age at onset > 50 years	Development of symptoms or findings beginning aged >=50 years
2. New headache	New onset, or new type, of localized pains in the head
3. Temporal artery abnormality	Temporal artery tenderness on palpation or decreased pulsation, unrelated to atherosclerosis of cervical arteries
4. Increased ESR	ESR>50 mm in first hour by Westergren method
5. Abnormal artery biopsy	Biopsy specimen with artery Showing vasculitis characterized by a predominance of mononuclear infiltration or granulomatous inflammation

Diagnosis of GCA requires at least three of five criteria to be present. The presence of any three or more criteria gives a sensitivity of 93.5% and specificity of 91.2% [5].

Inflammatory markers such as ESR and C-reactive protein (CRP) aid in the diagnosis of PMR and GCA and can also be used to monitor disease activity, however normal ESR and CRP results do not rule out GCA.

Temporal artery biopsy (TAB) is the "gold standard" for diagnosis of GCA. A TAB is considered to be positive if there is interruption of the internal elastic laminae with infiltration of mononuclear cells into the arterial wall. Multinucleated giant cells are seen, but are not required for diagnosis. GCA affects vessels focally and segmentally, resulting in areas of inflammatory vasculitis lesions around areas of normal artery.

High-resolution colour Doppler ultrasonography (CDUS) can show both the vessel wall and the lumen, and may show early vessel wall damage while the lumen is still unaffected. The inflamed temporal arteries in GCA have a concentric hypoechogenic mural thickening, called a "halo", which is a result of inflammatory vessel wall oedema. The "halo" is very specific for GCA, and less specific signs are stenoses and occlusions.

Inflammation of the aorta and its branches may occur, although symptoms may occur years after the initial diagnosis. MRI can aid in diagnosing early large vessel vasculitis in GCA. Typical changes in inflamed vessels include thickening and oedema of the vessel wall, which precede the development of stenoses or aneurysms, detected by angiography. Magnetic resonance angiography is used to show alterations in the vessel lumen, such as stenoses and aneurysms. MRI and CT are useful in evaluating deep, large vessels such as the thoracic and the abdominal aorta, which are frequently involved in GCA. PET may be used to confirm the diagnosis of large vessel GCA because of its ability to identify inflammatory cell infiltration of the vessel wall, which is one of the earliest signs of large vessel vasculitis.

Management includes high doses of GCS. Glucocorticosteroids are the main treatment in GCA because of their ability to quickly control inflammatory symptoms and prevent most ischemic manifestations, including loss of vision.

In patients with GCA, without severe ischemic complications, an initial dose of prednisone or its equivalent of 40 mg/day (or 0.7 mg/kg) as a single or divided dose for 3-4 weeks is recommended. In patients with GCA who present with visual ischemic complications or other severe ischemic manifestations, such as cerebrovascular accidents or large artery stenosis of the extremities resulting in occlusion (limb claudication) of recent onset, an initial prednisone dose of 60 mg/day is needed. A 3-day course of intravenous methylprednisolone pulses a 1000 mg may result in quicker GCS tapering, a lower median dose at each visit and fewer relapses. The use of GCS has decreased the frequency of severe visual ischemic complications in patients with GCA. Data reveals that it is not the total dose but the time from onset of symptoms to first administration of GCS that is predictive of improvement in visual loss. Once visual loss is established, the prognosis for significant visual recovery in patients with GCA despite GCS therapy is poor.

Other GCA symptoms usually begin to improve within 24-72 h after the start of GCS therapy. Normalization of routine laboratory parameters of inflammation (CRP, and then ESR) occurs 2-4 weeks after starting treatment. The GCS dose can be gradually tapered. Prednisone is reduced by 5 mg every 2-4 weeks to 25 mg. It can then be reduced by 2.5 mg every 2-4 weeks until the dose 10 mg, and later by about 1 mg every month. The duration of GCS therapy in GCA is variable, and as relapses often occur, may last for 2-4 years, and sometimes cannot be stopped.

Immunosuppressive agents may be used in large vessel vasculitis as adjunctive treatment. Glucocorticoid-sparing drugs such as MTX or azathioprine should be considered in patients with GCA with severe glucocorticoid-related side effects and/or in patients who need prolonged glucocorticoid therapy due to disease relapse.

The IL-6 blocker tocilizumab (a humanized anti-IL-6 receptor monoclonal antibody) is be effective.

Aspirin may be used for the adjuvant treatment of patients with GCA. Bone protection treatment should be used in patients with GCA as long-term GCS therapy induces bone loss. Drugs that restore balanced bone cell activity, by directly decreasing the rate of osteoblast apoptosis (such as cyclical parathyroid hormone) or by increasing the rate of osteoclast apoptosis (such as bisphosphonates), may be useful in the management of patients with GCA receiving lon-term GCS therapy.

Polymyalgia Rheumatica (PMR)

PMR is characterized by pain and stiffness of the neck, shoulders, and pelvic girdle. The musculoskeletal symptoms are bilateral and symmetric. Morning stiffness is the predominant feature.

PMR affects the middle aged and elderly. The response to small doses of GCS is very quick. PMR is often accompanied with GCA. Management includes low doses of GCS (10-20 mg prednisone per day).

The ACR and EULAR in 2012 gives classification criteria for PMR [6]. According to the criteria, patients with new-onset bilateral shoulder pain and stiffness not explained by other diseases who are 50 years of age and older, and have elevated inflammatory markers such as CRP and ESR and have the following features:

Morning stiffness of greater than 45 minutes (2 points)

Hip pain/limited range of motion (1 point)

Normal rheumatoid factor and/or anticitrullinated protein antibody (2 points)

And absence of peripheral joint pain (1 point).

To diagnose polymyalgia rheumatica a total score has to be greater than or equal to four and it has 68% sensitivity and 78% specificity [6].

The response to GCS is rapid, with complete or nearly complete improvement within a few days. Some patients with PMR require an increase of dosage of prednisone to 30 mg/day. Higher initial GCS doses and faster tapering were significant predictors of relapses. The presence of symptoms, and an ESR or CRP value, can be used to monitor GCS doses. One to two years of treatment is usually required. However, some patients may require low doses of GCS for several years.

The risk of vertebral fractures is five times greater among women with PMR. Older age at diagnosis, a cumulative dose of prednisone of at least 2 g, and female sex independently increased the risk of adverse events.

BMD at the lumbar spine and hip should be performed when patients are starting GCS. If normal, BMD should be repeated after 12 months of GCS treatment. Bisphosphonates are indicated in patients with abnormal bone mineral density.

Interleukin-6 is an important molecule in the pathogenesis of PMR, and therefore IL-6 inhibition with tocilizumab (humanized monoclonal antibody to sIL-6R) may be a target.

MEDIUM VESSEL VASCULITIS (MVV)

Vasculitis affecting mostly medium arteries such as the main visceral arteries and their branches. Inflammatory aneurysms and stenoses are common. The onset of inflammation in MVV is more acute and necrotizing than the onset of inflammation in LVV.

Polyarteritis nodosa (PAN) is necrotizing arteritis of medium or small arteries.

In PAN small and medium-sized artery inflammation involve the skin, kidneys, peripheral nerves, muscles, and gut in patients of all ages, including children and the elderly, but predominates in patients between 40-60 years old, sex ratio – men: women = 2: 1.

The causes of primary or secondary PAN can be distinguished, since PAN can be the consequence of HBV infection and sometimes other etiological agents, like human immunodeficiency virus or, more controversially, hepatitis C virus. Among the vasculitides, PAN is now less common than in the past for reason of vaccination against HBV virus.

Clinical features include non-specific symptoms such as fever, chills, fatigue, anorexia, weight loss, malaise, skin involvement (palpable purpura, necrotic lesions, infarct of digital tips, livedo reticularis), myalgia, arthralgia and arthritis, peripheral mono/polyneuropathy (mononeuritis multiplex), renal involvement (renal sediment abnormality [red blood cells and red blood casts, proteinuria], renal insufficiency, hypertension), gut involvement (abdominal pain, infarction, hemorrhage, liver function abnormalities) and cardiac involvement (heart failure).

1990 Criteria for the Classification of Polyarteritis Nodosa [7]:

1. Weight loss >4 kg. Loss of 4 kg or more of body weight since illness began, not due to dieting or other factors.
2. Livedo reticularis – Mottled reticular pattern over the skin of portions of the extremities or torso.
3. Testicular pain or tenderness – Pain or tenderness of the testicles, not due to infection, trauma or other causes.
4. Myalgias, weakness or polyneuropathy – Diffuse myalgias (excluding shoulder and hip girdle) or weakness of muscles or tenderness of leg muscles.
5. Mononeuropathy or polyneuropathy – Development of mononeuropathy, multiple mononeuropathies, or polyneuropathy.
6. Diastolic BP>90 mmHg – Development of hypertension with the diastolic BP higher than 90 mmHg.
7. Elevated BUN or creatinine – Elevation of BUN>40 mg/dl or creatinine >1.5 mg/dl, not due to dehydration or obstruction.
8. Hepatitis B virus – presence of hepatitis B surface antigen or antibody in serum.
9. Arteriographic abnormality – Arteriogram showing aneurysms or occlusions of the visceral arteries, not due to arteriosclerosis, fibromuscular dysplasia, or other noninflammatory causes.
10. Biopsy of small or medium-sized artery containing – Histologic changes showing the presence of granulocytes or granulocytes and mononuclear leucocytes in the artery wall.

Diagnosis of polyarteritis nodosa **requires** at least three of ten criteria to be present. The presence of any three or more criteria gives a sensitivity of 82.2% and specificity of 86.6% [7].

Management includes high doses of GCS, cyclophosphamide and azathioprine.

In chronic hepatitis B, glucocorticoids and immunosuppressive drugs increase viral replication, even though they have proved to be useful against the symptoms of vasculitis. Used long term they enhance chronic HBV infection and aid cirrhosis progression, which may later cause hepatocellular carcinomas.

Therefore, the duration of glucocorticoid use must be short to rapidly control the most severe life-threatening manifestations of PAN. GCS should be abruptly stopped after 2-4 weeks to increase immunological clearance of HBV-infected hepatocytes and aid HBeAg to anti-HBeAb seroconversion. Later, treatment consists of plasma exchange to clear circulating immune complexes and is used until HBeAg to anti-HBeAg seroconversion is achieved. Antiviral agents must also be given to control viral replication as the final part of treatment, beginning in the first weeks. Currently, a combination of antiviral agents (*e.g.*, tenofovir and/or entecavir) is best, using interferon alpha 2b, lamivudine and/or other newer antiviral drugs.

Treatment for other virus-related PAN is also a combination of short courses of GCS therapy and antiviral agents, together with plasma exchange when symptoms are severe.

Treatment of non-viral PAN.

Methylprednisolone pulses (usually 7.5 to 15 mg/kg intravenously over 60 min repeated at 24 h intervals for 1-3 days) are used at the start of treatment. Oral GCS are given at a dose of 1 mg/kg/day of prednisone-equivalent, usually as a single morning dose. After of 3-4 weeks of the full dose, the GCS dose should be tapered and, in the absence of relapse, GCS can be stopped after 9-12 months.

CYC can be given orally and continuously or using intravenous bolus. Initial pulse dose of CYC range from 0.5 g to 1.2 g at intervals of 2 weeks initially, then every to 3 weeks to 1 month maximum. The oral CYC dose is 2 mg/kg/day, usually with a maximum of 200 mg/day. Once remission is achieved with CYC, patients can be switched to a less toxic immunosuppressive agent for maintenance, usually AZA (dose is 2 mg/kg/day or MTX to 25 mg orally or subcutaneously). The overall optimal duration of maintenance treatment is unknown.

Kawasaki Disease (KD) affects medium and small arteries. It is an acute febrile mucocutaneous and lymph node disease affecting children aged <5 years, mainly in Asians. Arteritis is also observed. Coronary arteries are often involved. Death is observed in 2% of children due to complications such as rupture of coronary arteries.

American Heart Association diagnostic criteria for Kawasaki disease [8]:

Fever of at least 5 days' duration and

Presence of four of the following main features:

1. Changes in extremities
2. Polymorphous exanthema
3. Bilateral conjunctival injection
4. Changes in the lips and oral cavity
5. Cervical lymphadenopathy

Patients with fever and fewer than four main clinical features can be diagnosed as having Kawasaki disease when coronary artery disease is detected by two-dimentional echocardiography or coronary angiography.

Exclusion of other similar diseases such as measles, scarlet fever, drug reactions, Stevens-Johnson syndrome, other febrile viral exanthems, Rocky Mountain spotted fever, staphylococcal scarlet skin syndrome, toxic shock syndrome, juvenile rheumatoid arthritis, leptospirosis and mercury poisoning [8].

Management includes IVIG and aspirin. Currently, the recommended therapy in the acute phase of KD is one infusion of IVIG (2g/kg/12-24 h) plus oral aspirin (30-50 mg) divided three times daily administered within the first 10 days of disease. After the fever has subsided the aspirin dose can be reduced to 3-5 mg/kg once a day for 6-8 weeks from onset. If coronary artery changes (eclasia or aneurysms) remain, low dose aspirin (3-5 mg/kg/day) should be continued until the changes regress.

SMALL VESSEL VASCULITIS (SVV)

Affects small vessels, including small intraparenchymal arteries, arterioles, capillaries, and venules. Medium arteries and veins may also be affected.

ANCA-associated Vasculitis (AAV) – Necrotizing vasculitis, with few or no immune deposits, mostly affecting small vessels.

Antineutrophil Cytoplasmic Antibodies (ANCA) are circulating autoantibodies directed against the cytoplasmic parts of neutrophils and monocytes. Two ANCA patterns can be seen by indirect immunofluorescence: the cytoplasmic (c-ANCA) and the perinuclear (p-ANCA) patterns; c-ANCA is associated with antibodies reacting with the 29-30 kDa elastinolytic enzyme, serine proteinase 3 (PR3). This is composed of 229 amino acids and found in the azurophilic granules of neutrophils and monocytes, but p-ANCA pattern is associated with antibodies to myeloperoxidase (MPO), a 140 kDa heterodymeric enzyme also associated with the antimicrobial properties of neutrophils. ANCA associated with primary small vessel systemic necrotizing vasculitis target lysosomal enzymes such as proteinase 3 and myeloperoxidase. ANCA are very strongly expressed in drug-induced syndromes, *e.g.* drug-induced lupus-like syndrome and drug-induced vasculitis.

Microscopic Polyangiitis (MPA) – Necrotizing vasculitis, with few or no immune deposits, affecting mostly small vessels (*i.e.*, capillaries, venules, or arterioles). Necrotizing arteritis involving small and medium arteries may also be present. Necrotizing glomerulonephritis is very common. Pulmonary capillaritis often occurs.

EPIDEMIOLOGY

MPA has been reported worldwide and can affect all racial groups, but is predominant in Caucasians. There is a slighty more male predominance than female, with the male to female ratio from 1.1 to 1.8. The average age at onset is about 50 years. The total annual incidence is estimated at 3-24 per million population, and the prevalence at 25-94 per million population [9].

CLINICAL FEATURES

Clinical features include myalgias, arthritis, rapidly progressive glomerulonephritis, microscopic haematuria with proteinuria also pulmonary manifestation in form of diffuse alveolar haemorrhage (caused by pulmonary capillaritis). Pulmonary-renal syndrome may occur as well. Other symptoms include pulmonary haemorrhage, characterized by dyspnoea and anaemia, and may progress to respiratory distress syndrome [10]. Intestinal lung fibrosis is a rare manifestation of MPA.

Skin lesions such as maculopapular purpuric lesions of the lower limbs are found in half of patients with MPA. Other lesions are vesicles, necrosis, ulcerations, nodules, splinter haemorrhages, livedo reticularis, hand and/or finger erythema, facial oedema and mouth ulcers. On histology, leucocytoclastic vasculitis of the small vessels of the dermis is observed.

Mononeuritis multiplex affects two-thirds of patients with peripheral nervous system involvement, followed by symmetric polyneuropathy. CNS involvement and cranial neuropathies have been reported in around 10% of patients.

Abdominal pain is present in up to 50% of patients. Sometimes bleeding or more severe small intestine or large bowel ischaemia, ulceration or perforations may occur.

Cardiovascular complications such as heart failure, pericarditis, myocardial infarction are rare.

Ocular manifestations such as eyelid inflammation, retinal cotton-wool spots, retinal vasculitis and choroiditis are rare.

LABORATORY FINDINGS

There is no specific laboratory test for diagnosing MPA. ANCA are detected in 60-80% of patients with MPA. The majority of ANCA detected are pANCA anti-MPO, also anti-PR3.

In patients with renal involvement microscopic haematuria is observed and shows an active glomerulonephritis. Proteinuria can be found in >90% of patients, but is usually <3.5 g per 24 h.

Renal histology is characterized by the presence of focal segmental thrombosing and necrotizing glomerulonephritis. Extracapillary crescents are present and involve more than 60% of the glomeruli.

PATHOGENESIS

Anti-MPO pANCA have a direct pathogenic role, which are supported by animal models [11].

Modifications in the Fc gamma receptor, present in neutrophils, have also been involved in the pathogenesis of the disease [12].

Epigenetic and genetic factors may have an influence on the pathogenesis and severity of the disease [12]. A genome-wide association study found a genetic influence of HLA-DQ in MPO-ANCA disease [13].

Granulomatosis with Polyangiitis (GPA) – Necrotizing granulomatous inflammation involving the upper and lower respiratory tract, and necrotizing vasculitis affecting mostly small to medium vessels (*e.g.*, capillaries, venules, arterioles, arteries and veins). Necrotizing glomerulonephritis, ocular vasculitis, pulmonary capillaritis with hemorrhage and granulomatous and nongranulomatous extravascular inflammation are common. CHCC 2012 replaced "Wegener's granulomatosis" with "granulomatosis with polyangiitis (Wegener's)" [1]. Limited expressions, especially in the upper or lower respiratory tract, or the eye may occur.

GPA occurs in patients between 30-50 years old, sex ratio = men: women = 1: 1. Aseptic inflammation leads to necrosis, granuloma formation and vasculitis of the upper and lower respiratory tracts. Glomerulonephritis may develop in 75% of patients. Destructive inflammatory lesions affect the eyes, ears, nose, trachea, bronchi and lungs. Renal disease occurs primarily in the form of glomerulonephritis and vasculitis. Clinical feature include: sinusitis, oral ulcers, otitis media, hemoptysis, active urinary sediment. Musculoskeletal features are common. About 25% of cases may have peripheral or central nervous system disease. Morbidity results mostly from airway, renal, auditory and ocular disease. c-ANCA – specificity marker for GPA is present in about 98% of patients.

CLINICAL MANIFESTATIONS

Constitutional symptoms such as fever, weight loss and fatigue may occur in 30 – 80% of patients [14].

Musculoskeletal symptoms are common, with non-deforming polyarthritis affecting medium- and large-size joints in two-thirds of patients [14].

Granulomatous ear, nose and throat lesions may be present in three-quarters of patients, with rhinitis, sinusitis, chronic otitis media, saddle-nose deformity and nasal septum perforation.

Hearing loss may occur (conductive and sensorineural) due to inflammation of middle ear, dysfunction of the Eustachian tube or cochlear artery vasculitis. Oral manifestations are ulcerative stomatitis or hyperplastic gingivitis. Laryngeal involvement can cause hoarseness and lead to subglottic stenosis in up to 15% of cases [15].

Two-thirds of patients have pulmonary involvement, with bilateral parenchymal nodules, cavitated in half of the cases, and/or alveolar hemorrhage in 10-20% of patients [15].

Rapidly progressive glomerulonephritis, also called necrotizing crescentic glomerulonephritis or pauci-immune glomerulonephritis, is the third main manifestation of GPA, present in 40-100% of patients.

Peripheral nervous system involvement occurs in one-third of patients, mainly present as mononeuritis multiplex (79% of the patients with peripheral neuropathy), then sensorimotor polyneuropathy. Central nervous system involvement is less common and can be seen in 6-13% of patients, usually later in the course of the disease.

Skin lesions occur in 10-50% of patients, with palpable purpura of the legs and feet. Necrotic papules on the extensor surfaces of the limbs, nodules or extensive and painful cutaneous ulcerations are less common.

Eye involvement, mainly episcleritis, is also frequent in GPA. Orbital granuloma or pseudo-tumor (which constitutes 15% of the eye involvement) may compress important muscles or nerves.

Gastrointestinal involvement is uncommon and cardiac manifestations are reported with a frequency 3.3% [16].

Histology

Histological confirmation should be performed when there is a suspicion of kidney involvement.

Nasal and/or sinus biopsy is easy to perform, but only 20-50% of such biopsies contribute to diagnosis.

Cutaneous biopsy often shows small vessel leucocytoclastic vasculitis.

Bronchoscopy with bronchoalveolar fluid examination can confirm alveolar haemorrhage and rule out suspicion of infection. Surgical biopsy of lung nodules show necrotizing vasculitis in up to 60% of cases.

Patogenesis of GPA

The etiopathogenesis of GPA remain unknown. Studies have shown a genetic predisposition in GPA where HLA-DPB1 is over-represented [17]. A genom-wide association study has provided evidence for the association of PR3-ANCA disease and *SERPINA1* and *PRTN3*. *SERPINA1* encodes alpha-1 antitrypsin, a serine protease which has PR3 as one of its substrates, and *PRTN3* encodes PR3 [13]. Staphylococcus aureus cross-react with the autoantigen (cPR3).

EPIDEMIOLOGY

The incidence of GPA ranges from 2 to 12 per million population and the prevalence from 24 to 157 per million people [9]. GPA is more frequent in northern rather than southern European countries.

There is no gender predominance in GPA and the peak incidence is in the fourth to sixth decade of life [14].

American College of Rheumatology classification criteria for granulomatosis with polyangiitis (Wegener's) [18]:

CRITERION	DEFINITION
1. Nasal or oral inflammation	Development of painful or painless oral ulcers or purulent or bloody nasal discharge
2. Abnormal chest radiograph	Chest radiograph showing the presence of nodules, fixed infiltrates or cavities
3. Urinary sediment	Microhaematuria (>5 red cells per high power field) or red cell casts in urinary sediment
4. Granulomatous inflammation on biopsy	Histological changes showing granulomatous inflammation within the wall of an artery or in the perivascular or extracascular area (artery or arteriole)

Diagnosis of granulomatosis with polyangiitis (Weneger's) requires two of four criteria to be present and gives a sensitivity of 88.2% and specificity of 92.0% [18].

BVAS (Birmingham Vasvulitis Activity Score) currently used to assess disease activity. BVAS assesses 66 disease symptoms, classified into 9 main modules which are divided into different organs and systems. It also has a prognostic value based on number of points.

BVAS – Birmingham Vasculitis Activity Score (version 3) [19]:

1. GENERAL

Myalgia

Arthralgia/arthritis

Fever ≥ 38°C

Weight loss ≥ 2 kg

2. CUTANEOUS

Infarct

Purpura

Ulcer

Gangrene

Other skin vasculitis

3. MUCOUS MEMBRANES/EYES

Mouth ulcers

Genital ulcers

Adnexal inflammation

Significant proptosis

Scleritis/Episcleritis

Conjuctivitis/Blepharitis/Keratitis

Blurred vision

Sudden visual loss

Uveitis

Retinal changes (vasculitis/thrombosis/exudates/haemorrage)

4. ENT (Ear, Nose and Throat)

Bloody nasal discharge/crusts/ulcers/granuloma

Paranasal sinus involvement

Subglottic stenosis

Conductive hearing loss

Sensorineural hearing loss

5. CHEST

Wheeze

Nodules or cavities

Pleural effusion/ pleurisy

Infiltrate

Massive haemoptysis /alveolar haemorrhage

Respiratory failure

6. CARDIOVASCULAR

Loss of pulses

Valvular heart disease

Pericarditis

Ischemic cardiac pain

Cardiomyopathy

Congestive cardiac failure

7. ABDOMINAL

Peritonitis

Bloody diarrhea

Ischemic abdominal pain

8. RENAL

Hypertension

Proteinuria>1+

Haematuria ≥ 10RBCs/hpf

Creatinine 125-249 u/L (1.41-2.82mg/dl)*

Creatinine 250-499 u/L (2.83-5.64 mg/dl)*

Creatinine ≥ 500 u/L (≥5.66 mg/dl)*

Rise in serum creatinine >30% or fall in creatinine clearance >25%

*can only be scored on the first assessment

9. NERVOUS SYSTEM

Headache

Meningitis

Organic confusion

Seizures (not hypertensive)

Cerebrovaclular accident

Spinal cord lesion

Cranial nerve palsy

Sensory peripheral neuropathy

Mononeuritis multiplex

10. OTHER

Major items highlighted

Immunosupressive therapy is very effective, but is associated with serious complications. Cycloophosphamide (CYC) for six months followed by azathioprine (AZA) for 12 months is as effective as one course of rituximab (375 mg/m^2 × 4), which in 2011 was approved by FDA in combination with GCS for the treatment of GPA and MPA. Rituximab is better for patients who want to preserve their fertility. CYC is very important in the treatment of GPA/MPA in patients with rapidly progressive glomerulonephritis with creatinine levels >4.0 mg/dl, alveolar hemorrhage requiring mechanical ventilation, past adverse events specific to rituximab, and active disease despite rituximab therapy.

Eosinophilic Granulomatosis with Polyangiitis (EGPA) – is a disease characterised by pulmonary and systemic small vessel vasculitis, extravascular granulomas and hypereosinophilia, which occurs in people with a history of late-onset asthma and allergic rhinitis. There are three major histopathological criteria, 1. tissue infiltration by eosinophils, 2. necrotizing vasculitis and 3. extravascular granulomas [20]. Nasal polyps are common. The name "Churg-Strauss syndrome" was changed to "EPGA". Granulomatous and nongranulomatous extravascular inflammation, such as nongranulomatous eosinophil-rich inflammation of lungs, myocardium, and gastrointestinal tract, is common.

EGPA occurs in patients between 40 to 60 years old. EGPA annual incidence is between 0 and 4 per million population and prevalence is between 7 and 22 per million population [9]. The mean age at diagnosis of EGPA is around 45-50 years, with a male to female ratio of about 1.

Clinical features: presence of atopic history, asthma and/or allergic rhinitis, constitutional symptoms: fever, weight loss, multi system involvement, including pulmonary infiltrates, mono/polyneuropathy, mononeuritis multiplex, purpura and nodules, eosinophilia. Systemic vasculitis occurs 4-9 years after the onset of asthma, with latency of 30 years.

General symptoms are fever or weight loss.

Arthralgias are frequent, but arthritis is rare, and joint deformity and radiological erosions do not occur with predominance in large joints. Myalgia is present in half of patients.

Asthma is a main feature of EPGA, but has a late onset at around the age of 35 years. The severity and frequency of the asthmatic attacks increase until the onset of vasculitis. Chest radiographs are abnormal and 38-77% of patients have transient pulmonary infiltrates, in contrast to GPA.

Maxillary sinusitis is common and 70% of patients have a history of allergic rhinitis and sinus polyposis.

Peripheral neuropathy usually mononeuritis multiplex is found in 45-75% of patients. CNS involvement is rare and occur in 5 -10% of patients and includes strokes and pachymeningitis.

Cutaneous lesions such as purpura is seen in half of cases and subcutaneous nodules in 30%. Skin biopsies show extravascular and eosinophilic granulomas. Other cutaneous manifestations include Raynaud's phenomenon, livedo reticularis, urticarial lesions, patchy skin necrosis, infiltrated papules, vesicles or bullae and toe or finger ischaemia.

Cardiac involvement is common in EGPA and it is a major cause of death. It is present in 17% using and 92% in post mortem studies. Cardiac features include pericarditis, myocarditis, arrhythmias and more rarely angina pectoris, myocardial infarction and sudden death.

Gastrointestinal symptoms including abdominal pain, diarrhea and bleeding occur in 30-60% of patients. Bowel perforation is the most severe GI complication and is one of the major causes of death.

Renal disease is uncommon in EGPA and it is usually found in <25% of patients. The glomerular lesion is focal segmental glomerulonephritis with necrotizing features including crescents. Kidney disease is less severe and rarely causing renal failure.

EGPA is associated with anti-MPO pANCA, but only 25-40% of patients with EGPA are ANCA-positive. In these patients, there is an increased frequency of renal involvement, constitutional symptoms, purpura, alveolar haemorrhage, mononeuritis multiplex and CNS involvement.

Eosinophilia is present in active untreated disease and often > 1500/mm^3 (97% of patients). Serun IgE is increased in more than 75% of patients.

Histological features include infiltration by eosinophils, necrotizing vasculitis and extravascular granulomas.

The pathophysiology of EGPA include the pathogenic role of T helper type 2 lymphocytes in asthma, eosinophils infiltrating tissues, and anti-MPO-ANCA. The association of the disease with HLA-DRB4 is very important [21].

Desentisation and vaccination is a potential triggering factors for the development of EGPA.

American College of Rheumatology classification criteria for Churg-Strauss syndrome [22]:

CRITERION	DEFINITION
1. Asthma	History of wheezing or diffuse high-pitched rales on expiration
2. Eosinophilia	Eosinophilia >10% on white cell differential count
3. Mononeuropathy or polyneuropathy	Development of mononeuropathy, multiple mononeuropathies or polyneuropathy (ie, glove/stocking distribution) attributable to systemic vasculitis
4. Pulmonary infiltrates, non-fixed	Migratory or transient pulmonary infiltrates on radiographs (not including fixed infiltrates), attributable to a systemic vasculitis
5. Paranasal sinus abnormality	History of acute or chronic paranasal sinus pain or tenderness or radiographic opacification of the paranasal sinuses
6. Extravascular eosinophils	Biopsy including artery, arteriole or venule showing accumulations of eosinophils in extravascular areas

Churg-Strauss syndrome is diagnosed if at least four of these six criteria are present. The presence of any four or more criteria gives a sensitivity of 85,0% and specificity of 99.7% [22].

Management includes high doses of GCS, CYC and AZA in serious cases.

INDUCTION THERAPY

Regimen for MPA and EGPA with poor prognostic factors and systemic/severe forms of GPA.

All patients should receive an induction regimen based on the combination of glucocorticoids (GCS) and an immunosuppressant agent, with cyclophosphamide

(CYC) or rituximab (RTX) as first choice [23].

Methylprednisolone pulses (usually 7.5-15 mg/kg intravenously over 60 min repeated at 24h intervals for 1-3 days). Oral GCS are given at a dose of 1mg/kg/day of prednisone-equivalent (usually as a single morning dose). After 3 – 4 weeks of the full dose, the GCS dose should be tapered and, in the absence of relapse, GCS can be stoped after 9 – 18 months [23].

CYC, an alkylating immunosuppressant agent, can be given orally and continuously or using an intravenous bolus.

The CYC dose intravenously ranges from 0.5 to 1.2 g at intervals of 2 weeks initially, then every 3 weeks to 1 month maximum. The oral CYC dose is 2mg/kg/day usually with a maximum of 200 mg/day [23].

Rituximab (RTX) a genetically engineered chimeric murine/human IgG1k monoclonal antibody directed against CD20 antigen expressed on the surface of B lymphocytes is an equally effective alternative treatment at 1 g every 2 weeks for a total of two injections.

Regimen for MPA or EGPA without poor prognostic factors and for localized early systemic forms of GPA.

Treatment with GCS alone – started orally at a dose of 1 mg/kg/day of prednisolone and after 3-4 weeks of the full dose, the GCS should be tapered [23].

Maintenance Treatment

Once remission is achieved with CYC, patients can be switched to a less toxic immunosuppressant agent for maintenance, such as AZA or MTX. The AZA dose is 2 mg/kg/day and the MTX dose is 0.3 mg/kg, delivered once weekly, up to 25 mg/week, orally or subcutaneously [23].

Immune complex small vessel vasculitis is vasculitis of vessel wall deposits of immunoglobulin and/or complement, affecting small vessels (*i.e.*, capillaries, venules, arterioles, and small arteries). Glomerulonephritis is frequent. Immune complex vasculitis can appear after hepatitis C virus-associated cryoglobulinemic vasculitis or as a vasculitis associated with systemic disease (*e.g.*, lupus vasculitis or rheumatoid vasculitis).

Anti-Glomerular Basement Membrane (anti-GBM) Disease is a vasculitis affecting glomerular capillaries, pulmonary capillaries, or both, with basement membrane deposition of anti-basement membrane autoantibodies. Lung involvement causes pulmonary hemorrhage, and renal involvement causes glomerulonephritis with necrosis and crescents. The name "Goodpasture's syndrome" has been used in the past for combined pulmonary and renal expression of anti-GBM disease.

Cryoglobulinemic Vasculitis (CV) is vasculitis with cryoglobulin immune deposits affecting small vessels (predominantly capillaries, venules, or arterioles) and associated with cryoglobulins in serum. Skin, glomeruli, and peripheral nerves are often involved. The term "idiopathic" or "essential" is used as to indicate that the etiology of CV is unknown.

IGA VASCULITIS (IGAV)

It is vasculitis with IgA1-dominant immune deposits, affecting small vessels. IgAV usually involves the skin (purpura over areas of the buttocks and lower extremities) and gastrointestinal tract (abdominal pain and bloody diarrhea) and frequently causes arthritis. Glomerulonephritis mimicking IgA nephropathy. The name "Henoch-Schnlein purpura" was changed to IgAV due to abnormal IgA deposits in vessel walls. The onset of symptomatic IgAV is associated with an upper respiratory tract or gastrointestinal infection. IgAV is the most common vasculitis syndrome of childhood in patients 5-18 years old, with sex prevalence boys to girls = 1: 1. The spectrum of the clinical expression may vary from only minimal petechial rash to severe gastrointestinal, renal, neurological, pulmonary and joint disease.

American College of Rheumatology classification criteria for Henoch-Schonlein purpura [24]:

CRITERION	DEFINITION
1. Palpable purpura	Slightly raised purpuric rash over one or more areas of the skin not related to thrombocytopenia
2. Bowel angina	Diffuse abdominal pain worse after meals, or bowel ischaemia, usually bloody diarrhea
3. Age at onset <20 years	Development of first symptoms at age <=20 years
4. Wall granulocytes on biopsy	Histological changes showing granulocytes in the walls of arteries or venules

Henoch-Schonlein purpura is diagnosed if at least two of these four criteria are present. The presence of any two or more criteria gives a sensitivity of 87.1% and specificity of 87.7% [24].

Treatment GCS in serious cases also immunosuppressive agents.

VARIABLE VESSEL VASCULITIS (VVV)

It is vasculitis with involvement of any size (small, medium, and large) and type (arteries, veins, and capillaries) for *e.g.* Behcet's disease (BD) and Cogan's syndrome.

BD Vasculitis is vasculitis occurring in patients with BD that can affect arteries or veins. BD is characterized by recurrent oral and/or genital aphthous ulcers accompanied by cutaneous, ocular, articular, gastrointestinal, and/or central nervous system inflammatory lesions. Small vessel vasculitis, arteritis, arterial aneurysms, and venous and arterial thromboangiitis and thrombosis may occur. BD has a marked geographic distribution and is characterized by greatest prevalence in Turkey, Iran and Japan, occurring in patients between 20-35 years old, with sex prevalence men: women = 1: 1.

International Study Group diagnostic criteria for Behcet's disease [25]:

CRITERION	DEFINITION
Reccurent oral ulceration	Minor aphthous, major aphthous or herpetiform ulceration seen by physician or patient, which reccured at least three times in one 12-month period
Plus two of:	
1. Recurrent genital ulceration	Aphthous ulceration or scarring seen by the physician or patient
2. Eye lesions	Anterior uveitis, posterior uveitis or cells in vitreous on slip-lamp examination; or retinal vasculitis seen by ophthalmologist
3. Skin lesions	Erythema nodosum seen by physician or patient, pseudofolliculitis, or papulopustular lesions; or acneiform nodules seen by physician in postadolescent patients not receiving glucocorticoid treatment
4. Positive pathergy test	Read by physician at 24-48 h

A patient must have recurrent oral ulceration plus at least two of the other findings in absence of other clinical explanations (sensitivity 91%, specificity 96%) [25].

Management of BD depends on the clinical presentation and organ involved. Although colchicines, non-steroidal anti-inflammatory drugs and topical treatment with GCS are often enough for mucocutaneous and joint involvement, a more aggressive approach with immunosuppressive agents (MTX, AZA, CYC, ciclosporin A) is used for severe manifestations such as posterior uveitis, retinal vasculitis, vascular, neurological and gastrointestinal involvement.

COGAN'S SYNDROME is a rare disease, consisting of interstitial keratitis, audiovestibular symptoms and systemic manifestations in young people, with a median age at onset of 25 years.

The eye symptoms are photophobia, redness, and local irritation. The audiovestibular symptoms are partial or total hearing loss, vertigo, and ataxia. Some patients have weight loss, fever, lymphadenopathy, hepatosplenomegaly and rash. Aortitis,causing aneurysms and aortic insufficiency is a very serious manifestation of Cogan's syndrome.

Management is not established, the interstitial keratitis is treated by topical corticosteroids, audiovestibular symptoms with high doses of corticosteroids, vasculitis with high-dose corticosteroids along with cytotoxic drugs, methotrexate and ciclosporin.

REFERENCES

[1]   Jennette JC, Falk RJ, Bacon PA, *et al.* 2012 revised International Chapel Hill Consensus Conference Nomenclature of Vasculitides. Arthritis Rheum 2013; 65(1): 1-11.
[http://dx.doi.org/10.1002/art.37715] [PMID: 23045170]

[2]   Kerr GS. Takayasu's arteritis. Rheum Dis Clin North Am 1995; 21(4): 1041-58.
[PMID: 8592736]

[3]   Arend WP, Michel BA, Bloch DA, *et al.* The American College of Rheumatology 1990 criteria for the classification of Takayasu arteritis. Arthritis Rheum 1990; 33(8): 1129-34.
[http://dx.doi.org/10.1002/art.1780330811] [PMID: 1975175]

[4]   Gonzalez-Gay MA, Vazquez-Rodriguez TR, Lopez-Diaz MJ, *et al.* Epidemiology of giant cell arteritis and polymyalgia rheumatica. Arthritis Rheum 2009; 61(10): 1454-61.
[http://dx.doi.org/10.1002/art.24459] [PMID: 19790127]

[5]   Hunder GG, Bloch DA, Michel BA, *et al.* The American College of Rheumatology 1990 criteria for the classification of giant cell arteritis. Arthritis Rheum 1990; 33(8): 1122-8.
[http://dx.doi.org/10.1002/art.1780330810] [PMID: 2202311]

[6]   Dasgupta B, Cimmino MA, Kremers HM, *et al.* 2012 Provisional classification criteria for polymyalgia rheumatica: a European League Against Rheumatism/American College of Rheumatology collaborative initiative. Arthritis Rheum 2012; 64(4): 943-54.
[http://dx.doi.org/10.1002/art.34356] [PMID: 22389040]

[7]   Lightfoot RW Jr, Michel BA, Bloch DA, *et al.* The American College of Rheumatology 1990 criteria for the classification of polyarteritis nodosa. Arthritis Rheum 1990; 33(8): 1088-93.
[http://dx.doi.org/10.1002/art.1780330805] [PMID: 1975174]

[8]   Dajani AS, Taubert KA, Gerber MA, *et al.* Diagnosis and therapy of Kawasaki disease in children. Circulation 1993; 87(5): 1776-80.
[http://dx.doi.org/10.1161/01.CIR.87.5.1776] [PMID: 8491037]

[9]   Mohammad AJ, Jacobsson LT, Westman KWA, Sturfelt G, Segelmark M. Incidence and survival rates in Wegener's granulomatosis, microscopic polyangiitis, Churg-Strauss syndrome and polyarteritis nodosa. Rheumatology (Oxford) 2009; 48(12): 1560-5.
[http://dx.doi.org/10.1093/rheumatology/kep304] [PMID: 19797309]

[10]   Sourla E, Bagalas V, Tsioulis H, *et al.* Acute respiratory failure as primary manifestation of antineutrophil cytoplasmic antibodies-associated vasculitis. Clin Pract 2014; 4(2): 653-6.
[http://dx.doi.org/10.4081/cp.2014.653] [PMID: 25332763]

[11]   Xiao H, Heeringa P, Hu P, *et al.* Antineutrophil cytoplasmic autoantibodies specific for

myeloperoxidase cause glomerulonephritis and vasculitis in mice. J Clin Invest 2002; 110(7): 955-63.
[http://dx.doi.org/10.1172/JCI0215918] [PMID: 12370273]

[12] Jennette JC, Falk RJ, Gasim AH. Pathogenesis of antineutrophil cytoplasmic autoantibody vasculitis. Curr Opin Nephrol Hypertens 2011; 20(3): 263-70.
[http://dx.doi.org/10.1097/MNH.0b013e3283456731] [PMID: 21422922]

[13] Lyons PA, Rayner TF, Trivedi S, *et al.* Genetically distinct subsets within ANCA-associated vasculitis. N Engl J Med 2012; 367(3): 214-23.
[http://dx.doi.org/10.1056/NEJMoa1108735] [PMID: 22808956]

[14] Lynch JP III, Tazelaar H. Wegener granulomatosis (granulomatosis with polyangiitis): evolving concepts in treatment. Semin Respir Crit Care Med 2011; 32(3): 274-97.
[http://dx.doi.org/10.1055/s-0031-1279825] [PMID: 21674414]

[15] Hoffman GS, Kerr GS, Leavitt RY, *et al.* Wegener granulomatosis: an analysis of 158 patients. Ann Intern Med 1992; 116(6): 488-98.
[http://dx.doi.org/10.7326/0003-4819-116-6-488] [PMID: 1739240]

[16] McGeoch L, Carette S, Cuthbertson D, *et al.* Cardiac involvement in granulomatosis with polyangiitis. J Rheumatol 2015; 42(7): 1209-12.
[http://dx.doi.org/10.3899/jrheum.141513] [PMID: 25934819]

[17] Xie G, Roshandel D, Sherva R, *et al.* Association of granulomatosis with polyangiitis (Wegener's) with *HLA-DPB1*04* and *SEMA6A* gene variants: evidence from genome-wide analysis. Arthritis Rheum 2013; 65(9): 2457-68.
[http://dx.doi.org/10.1002/art.38036] [PMID: 23740775]

[18] Leavitt RY, Fauci AS, Bloch DA, *et al.* The American College of Rheumatology 1990 criteria for the classification of Wegener's granulomatosis. Arthritis Rheum 1990; 33(8): 1101-7.
[http://dx.doi.org/10.1002/art.1780330807] [PMID: 2202308]

[19] Mukhtyar C, Lee R, Brown D, *et al.* Modification and validation of the Birmingham Vasculitis Activity Score (version 3). Ann Rheum Dis 2009; 68(12): 1827-32.
[http://dx.doi.org/10.1136/ard.2008.101279] [PMID: 19054820]

[20] Pagnoux C. Churg-Strauss syndrome: evolving concepts. Discov Med 2010; 9(46): 243-52.
[PMID: 20350492]

[21] Vaglio A, Martorana D, Maggiore U, *et al.* HLA-DRB4 as a genetic risk factor for Churg-Strauss syndrome. Arthritis Rheum 2007; 56(9): 3159-66.
[http://dx.doi.org/10.1002/art.22834] [PMID: 17763415]

[22] Masi AT, Hunder GG, Lie JT, *et al.* The American College of Rheumatology 1990 criteria for the classification of Churg-Strauss syndrome (allergic granulomatosis and angiitis). Arthritis Rheum 1990; 33(8): 1094-100.
[http://dx.doi.org/10.1002/art.1780330806] [PMID: 2202307]

[23] Groh M, Pagnoux C, Baldini C, *et al.* Eosinophilic granulomatosis with polyangiitis (Churg-Strauss) (EGPA) Consensus Task Force recommendations for evaluation and management. Eur J Intern Med 2015; 26(7): 545-53.
[http://dx.doi.org/10.1016/j.ejim.2015.04.022] [PMID: 25971154]

[24] Mills JA, Michel BA, Bloch DA, *et al.* The American College of Rheumatology 1990 criteria for the classification of Henoch-Schönlein purpura. Arthritis Rheum 1990; 33(8): 1114-21.
[http://dx.doi.org/10.1002/art.1780330809] [PMID: 2202310]

[25] Criteria for diagnosis of Behçet's disease. Lancet 1990; 335(8697): 1078-80.
[PMID: 1970380]

CHAPTER 9

Gout

Abstract: Gout is an inflammatory disease caused by the deposition of monosodium urate (MSU) crystals in joints and other tissues. The formation of crystals is caused by hyperuricaemia, when serum uric acid (SUA) levels are >6.0 mg/dl (360 umol/L). Palpable deposits of MSU crystals are known as tophi and form around joints. The disease presents with episodes of joint inflammation. Renal lithiasis and formation of tophi in internal organs may also occur. Gout may induce disability, severe nephropathy and increases cardiovascular risk.

Uric acid is the final metabolite of purine metabolism in humans due to inactive urate oxidase (uricase). Hyperuricaemia may be caused by diet (*e.g.* alcohol, seafood, red meat), overproduction and undersecretion of urate. Gout may be primary and secondary. Primary gout may be associated with obesity, alcohol consumption, hypertension, type 2 diabetes and hypertrigliceridaemia. Secondary gout may be due to drugs (*e.g.* diuretics), in patients with nephropathy and myelolimphoproliferative diseases.

Gout is painful and a swollen red toe is characteristic (podagra). Attacks may be polyarticular in hand, wrist, ankle, knee.

Chronic urate arthropathy is destructive arthropathy with bone erosions and tophi.

The aim of the treatment of gout is to eliminate the urate crystals. The acute attacks must be treated with NSAIDs, GCS or colchicines; hyperuricaemia must be in the serum less than 6 mg/dl (0.36 mmol/L). IL-1 inhibitors may be used in patients with an inadequate response to standard drugs.

For urate lowering therapy was used xanthine oxidase inhibitors (allopurinol, febuxostat), uricosuric agents (probenecid, lesinurat) and uricase agents (pegloticase) were used.

Keywords: A swollen red toe, Allopuriniol, Bone erosions, Cardiovascular risk, Chronic urate arthropathy, Colchicines, Febuxostat, GCS, Gout, Hyperuricaemia, IL-1 inhibitors, Lesinurat, Monosodium urate (MSU) crystals, Nephropathy, NSAIDs, Pegloticase, Podagra, Probenecid, Purine metabolism, Renal lithiasis, Serum uric acid (SUA), The urate lowering therapy, Tophi, Urate oxidase (uricase), Uricase agents, Uricosuric agents, Xanthine oxidase inhibitors.

Małgorzata Wisłowska

INTRODUCTION

Gout is an inflammatory disease caused by the deposition of monosodium urate (MSU) crystals in joints and other tissues. The formation of crystals is caused by hyperuricaemia, and are formed when serum uric acid (SUA) levels are >6.0 mg/dl (360 umol/L) [1]. However, most patients with hyperuricaemia never have gout. Palpable deposits of MSU crystals are known as tophi and usually form around joints. The disease presents with episodes of joint inflammation. Renal lithiasis and formation of tophi in internal organs and other structures may also occur. Gout may induce disability and severe nephropathy and increases cardiovascular risk.

Gout is the most common form of inflammatory arthritis in men and its incidence and prevalence is rising in postmenopausal women. In Western countries gout affects 1-2% of adults, with a prevalence increasing with age, being 7% in men over 65 years and 3% in women over 85 years [2].

The presence of gout is associated with other co-morbidities, which may require modification of dietary and lifestyle habits and often drugs. Gout is also an independent risk factor for atherosclerotic cardiovascular disease [3].

ETIOPATHOLOGY

Common dysfunctional variants in ABCG2 gene are a major cause of early onset of gout. Uric acid is the final metabolite of purine metabolism. Purines are heterocyclic aromatic organic compounds, consisting of a pyrimidine ring bound to an imidazole ring. Uric acid is an acid with pH of 5.75. At a physiological pH of 7.4 in the extracellular compartment, 98% of uric acid is in the ionised form of urate. Because of the high concentration of sodium in the extracellular compartment, urate is present as MSU, with a solubility limit of 380 umol/L [4]. The risk of MSU crystal formation and precipitation is increased when the concentration is above this limit.

The levels of SUA depend on the balance between purine ingestion, synthesis and degradation. The ingestion of purine and/or urate is about 10% of the total pool of urate in the body. The synthesis of SUA is in the liver. The salvage pathways are a major source of nucleotides for synthesis of DNA, RNA and enzyme cofactors. Adenosine phosphoribosyltransferase and hypoxanthine-guanine phosphor-ribosyltransferase (HGPRT) are the enzymes involved in these salvage pathways and the end xanthine oxidase enzyme catalyses the oxidation of hypoxanthine to xanthine, and xanthine to uric acid.

The beginning of uric acid synthesis is the ribose-5-phosphate, a pentose derived from glycidic metabolism, converted to phosphoribosyl pyrophosphate (PRPP) and then to phosphoribosilamine, that will be transformed into inosine monophosphate (IMP). Adenosine monophosphate (AMP) and guanosine monophosphate (GMP) is derived, the purinic nucleotides used for DNA and RNA synthesis, and inosine that will be degraded into hypoxanthine and xanthine and finally, into uric acid. Hypoxanthine and guanine may enter in a salvage pathway, using HGPRT, an enzyme that reconverts these purines bases into their corresponding nucleotides. In a similar pathway, adenine phosphoribosyl-transferase (APRT) converts adenosine to AMP.

In humans urate oxidase (uricase), a hepatic enzyme, is inactive as a result of a non-sense mutation. Only animals which possess uricase can transform uric acid in a more soluble and more eliminable molecule: allantoin.

Urate is a breakdown product of the purine residues of nucleic acid, namely quinine and adenine. The pathway of the novo synthesis of the nucleic acid residues proceed *via* the key compounds 5-phosphoribosyl-1-pyrophosphate, and inosic acid. Inosic acid can either be converted into nucleic acid, or broken down through hypoxanthine and xanthine to form uric acid.

The whole pathway is controlled by feedback inhibition. Uric acid is not degraded in humans because there are no enzymes. 100% of uric acid is filtrated, 92-96% is reabsorbed and 8% is excreted.

The urate crystals are recognized by the innate immune system and cause an attacks. The molecules recognized by the innate immune system are called damage-associated molecular patterns (DAMPs) and include uric acid microcrystals. Recognition of DAMPs is mediated by germline-encoded molecules known as pattern recognition receptors (PRRFs). PRRs are expressed by many cell types, some of which are specialized effector cells of the immune system (*e.g.* neutrophils, macrophages, dendritic cells, lymphocytes). When PRRs are activated by DAMPs, effector cells containing the PRRs are triggered to perform their immune effector function immediately.

MSU crystals can activate the NLRP3-inflammasome, a multi molecular intracellular complex that converts pro-interleukin 1 and pro-IL-18 into their active forms [5], leading to gout inflammation [6]. MSU crystals activate IL-1beta of the gouty inflammatory response [6].

Defects of the enzymes involved in the salvage pathways may cause severe diseases, such as partial or total deficiency of HGPRT, which causes Lesch-Nyhan disease in boys.

Another cause of secondary hyperuricaemia is the raised activity of phosphoribosyl pyrophosphate synthetase, in which hyperuricaemia and gout are associated with renal overexcretion of uric acid and lithiasis.

The total amant of uric acid is about 1 gram and serum uric acid levels range from 0.1 to 0.4 mmols/L.

SUA levels depend on gender and age. Children have low SUA levels. At puberty SUA levels rise to the levels that will be maintained throughout life owing to a decrease in the renal clearance of urate, at least in women [2]; in men these levels rise slightly with age. Oestrogens are uricosuric so that hyperuricaemia will be lower in women up to menopause or end of hormonal substitution treatment [7].

Hyperuricaemia may be caused by:

• Diet (alcohol consumption, particularly beer, seafood and red meat). The consumption of some foods may be protective *e.g.* milk and yogurt;
• Overproduction of urate;
• Undersecretion of urate.

Gout may be primary (most are undersecretors, a few are overproducers) and secondary (undersecretion: *e.g.* renal failure, diuretic therapy). Overproduction: *e.g.* myeloproliferative diseases.

Excess uric acid may result from an increase in the amount of purines being degraded, either endogenously from tumours or haematological disorders like leukaemia or lymphomas, especially when treated, or in psoriasis [7].

Urate is poorly soluble and has to be transported across cell membranes. Different urate transporters such as URAT (urate transporter/channel) 1, and GLUT (glucose transporter) 9, two members of the family of organic anion transporters (OAT1 and OAT3) related to tubular secretion of urate for tubular secretion of urate and the main protein responsible for tubular reabsorption of urate [7].

Primary hyperuricaemic patients are characterized by increasing uricuria when hyperuricaemia increases, which is due to particular polymorphisms of the genes involved in the tubular transport of urate. The normal fractional excretion of urate is 7 – 10%, which represents the percentage of the filtrated urate which is finally excreted. Decreased fractional excretion of urate causes raised SUA levels which accompany the metabolic syndrome [7] – which is correctable by changing to a low caloric diet [7], - essential hypertension [7], decompensated heart failure [7], saturnine gout – which is correctable by lead chelation [7] – and alcohol consumption. Some drugs such as ciclosporin [7], low-dose aspirin [7], and diuretics also produce hyperuricaemia by reducing the fractional excretion of urate [7].

A third of the excretion of uric acid which is produced daily, is excreted *via* the intestines. Reduced interstinal excretion of urate is a possible cause of hyperuricaemia [7].

Gout may be classified as primary or secondary, depending on the presence or absence of an identified cause of hyperuricaemia.

Primary gout may be associated with other conditions, such as obesity, alcohol consumption, hypertension, type 2 diabetes and hypertrigliceridaemia.

Secondary gout may be due to drugs, such as diuretics, and drugs used in organ transplantation, mainly ciclosporin and tacrolimus.

Nephropathy is often found in association with gout. The presence of kidney stones is most common, occurring in 10-40% of patients, with a higher risk than for patients without gout. An association between hyperuricaemia and renal dysfunction has been observed [1].

Patients with hyperuricaemia and gout should be assessed for the presence of metabolic syndrome, which has a prevalence of 60-70%. The presence of metabolic syndrome may explain the presence of an increased cardiovascular risk in patients with hyperuricaemia, especially with gout [3].

CLINICAL FEATURES

Gout has three periods: asymptomatic hyperuricaemia, acute attacks with asymptomatic intervals and chronic gout.

Acute Gout

Acute gout is characterized by a rapid development of severe pain and swelling, with overlying erythema and tenderness that peaks within 6 -12 hours, often starting at night or in the early morning [8].

Gout is very painful and a swollen red toe in early acute gout is characteristic. Seventy percent of all acute attacks occur in the first metatarsophalangeal joint (MTP) (podagra). The attack may be precipitated by trauma, alcoholic excess, or current illness. The pain often starts at night and usually becomes extremely severe within a few hours. It is associated with joint swelling and red shiny skin. Desquamation of the skin often occurs. The toe returns to a normal state after a few days or weeks. Gout is also common in the hand, wrist, ankle and knee.

Attacks may be polyarticular involving two, three or more sites.

Less often, the disease starts in other joints: tarsal and subtalar joints, ankle, knee, wris and metacarpophalangeal or interphalangeal joints of the hand are frequently affected. Inflammation at the Achilles tendon insertion, of the olecranon bursae or patellar tendon is also common [9].

As the disease progresses without treatment, gouty attacks become more frequent, affect additional joints and become more polyarticular and persistent, leading to chronic gout. Gout at prosthetic joints has been reported [10, 11].

Chronic Gout

Chronic urate arthropathy is a late feature of neglected gout and is generally associated with palpable tophi. Evidence of chronic gouty changes in the bones include erosions and finger tophi, seen as shiny white deposits of urate which are visible through the skin. Tophi can be found as mases in different locations of the body. Narrowing of cartilage space is characteristically a late stage. The association of subchondral bone erosions, osteophytes and long preserved cartilage space is suggestive of urate arthropathy.

Chronic urate arthropathy is destructive arthropathy, due to urate infiltration of joints, is responsible for mechanical pain and permanent disability, with acute or subacute inflammatory episodes.

DIAGNOSIS

Identification of MSU crystals in synovial fluid samples from joints undergoing gouty attacks or from tophi leads to the diagnosis of gout [12].

Joint aspiration is useful in the diagnosis of gout or when there is a suspicion of gout. Ultrasonography should be used to aid arthrocentesis in difficult locations [13].

The technique of crystal detection and identification in synovial fluid is a simple procedure, a microscope allows detection and identification of MSU [14]. Definitive diagnosis of gout is based on joint aspiration and crystal identification.

2015 Gout Classification Criteria: An American College of Rheumatology/ European League Against Reumatism Collaborative Initiative [15]

Step 1: Entry criterion (only apply criteria below to those meeting this entry criterion). At least 1 episode of swelling, pain, or tenderness in a peripheral joint or bursa.

Step 2: Sufficient criterion (if met, can classify as gout without applying criteria below Presence of MSU crystals in a symptomatic joint or bursa (*i.e.* in synovial fluid) or tophus.

Step 3: Criteria (to be used if sufficient criterion not met).

CLINICAL

Pattern of joint/bursa involvement during symptomatic episode(s) ancle or mid-foot (as part of monoarticular or oligoarticular episode without involvement of the first metatarsophalangeal joint	1
Involvement of the first metatarsophalangealJoint (as part of monoarticular or oligoarticular episode)	2

Characteristics of Symptomatic Episode(s)

- Erythema overlying affected joint (patient-reported or physician- observed

One characteristic	1

- Can't bear touch or pressure to affected joint

Two characteristic	2

- Great difficulty with walking or inability to use affected joint

Three characteristics	3

Time Course of Episode(s)

Presence of >=2, irrespective or anti-inflammatory treatment:

- Time to maximal pain < 24 h One typical episode	3
- Resolution of symptoms in <= 14 days Recurrent typical episodes	2

- Complete resolution (to baseline level) between symptomatic episodes

Clinical evidence of tophus

Draining or chalk-like subcutaneous nodule under transparent skin, often with overlying vascularity, located in typical locations: joints, ears, olecranon bursae, finger pads, tendons (*e.g.* Achilles)

Present	4

LABORATORY

Serum urate: Measured by the uricase method.

Ideally should be scored at a time when the patient was not receiving urate-lowering treatment and it was > 4 weeks from the start of an episode (*i.e.* during the intercritical period); if practicable, retest under those conditions. The highest value irrespective of timing should be scored:

<4 mg/dL (0.24 mmol/L)	-4
6-8 mg/dL (0.36-<0.48 mmol/L)	2
8 -<10 mg/dL (0.48-<0.60 mmol/L)	3
>=10 mg/dL (>=0.60 mmol/L)	4

Synovial fluid analysis of a symptomatic episode.

Joint or bursa (should be assessed by a trained observer)

MSU negative	-2

IMAGING

Imaging evidence of urate deposition in symptomatic (ever) joint or bursa: ultrasound evidence of double-contour sign or DECT demonstrating urate deposition Present (either modality)	4
Imaging evidence of gout-related joint damage: conventional radiography of the hands and/or feet demonstrates at least 1 erosion Present	4

The maximum possible score in the final criteria is 23. A threshold score of ≥8 classifies an individual as having gout. The sensitivity and specificity of the criteria are high (92% and 89%, respectively) [15].

MANAGEMENT OF GOUT

Main aims of treatment are the treatment of acute attacks and the cure and the prevention of chronic disease. The final aim of the treatment of gout is to eliminate the urate crystals. Without crystals the possibility of joint inflammation disappears [8].

The goal is treating acute attacks early and effectively. In most cases, correcting hyperuricaemia either by determining a correctable cause or by using drugs. The aim is for the serum urate to be consistently less than 6 mg/dl (0.36 mmol/L). NSAIDs, GCS or colchicines may be used. Colchicine is used as prophylaxis between attacks. Colchicine 0.5 mg × 3 times on the first day of the attack, than

0.5 mg per day.

Innovative drugs, such as biological drugs acting as IL-1 inhibitors, in patients with inadequate response or contraindication/ intolerance to standard drugs.

All drugs indicated for an acute attack may be used alone or in combination with each other. The treatment can be maintained after symptoms lessen to avoid rebounds, generally at lower doses of a single drug.

Colchicine

Colchicine is an alkaloid derived from a plant, the Colchicum autumnale, and has been in use for the treatment of gout for a long time. Adverse effects are diarrhoea and vomiting.

Severe toxicity, with myelosuppression and myotoxicity, is uncommon and usually associated with high doses and prolonged use. It is seen in older patients with renal, hepatic or other comorbidities.

Continuation of a lower dose of colchicine – 0.5 mg twice a day is needed for 1-2 weeks to treat the attack, and for several months if a urate-lowering drug is added to prevent ultra-low-dose-induced flares.

NSAIDs

All NSAIDs given to treat acute attacks of gout have shown efficacy. Side effects including gastrointestinal, cardiovascular and renal systems.

Gouty attacks often occur in aged patients with comorbidities, in whom NSAIDs can be dangerous, especially in patients taking oral anticoagulants.

Glucocorticoids

A short course of systemic glucocorticoids (such as 30-35 mg of prednisone for 3-5 days with a rapid tapering off) [16] has been found effective. Recent ACR guidelines recommended starting treatment with oral prednisone 0.5 mg/kg per day with a duration of 5 – 10 days or 2 – 5 days of full doses, then tapering for 7 – 10 days and then stopping [16].

Short courses of GCS can be followed by a rebound attack of gout and co-administration of prophylactic doses of colchicine (0.5-1.0 mg/day) may be administered.

Intra-articular GCS are effective when large joints are affected. Intra-articular treatment of GCS could be used in combination with oral GCS, colchicine or an

NSAID [16].

Improvement has been observed after parenteral adrenocorticotropic hormone for patients unable to take oral anti-inflammatory drugs [16].

The Interleukin -1 Blockade

The role of IL-1 beta in gouty inflammation agents which block this cytokine may be used in serious cases.

Three agents are available:

1. Canakinumab,

2. Rilonacept (IL-Trap),

3. Anakinra.

The differences in clinical between these agents is their half-life, the longest being canakinumab (21-28 days), followed by rilonacept (34-57 h) and anacinra with a half-life of 4 – 6 h.

IL-1 blockade is a useful and selective treatment strategy for patients, who cannot tolerate standard treatments such as NSAIDs, colchicine or GCS. Current infection is a contraindication to the use of IL-1 blockers.

PREVENTION AND TREATMENT OF HYPERURICAEMIA

Correction and reversal of factors causing hyperuricaemia, *e.g.* regular alcohol intake (especially beer), high purine intake, obesity, diuretic therapy, suboptimal urine flow, hypertension, and/or use a urate lowering drug.

Correctable Factors Contributing to Hyperuricaemia

- Obesity

- Hypertriglyceridemia

- Regular alcohol consumption

- Diuretic therapy

- Inadequately controlled hypertension

- High dietary purine consumption

- Urine flow (<1 ml/min).

Prophylaxis of Urate Lowering Therapy Induces Gouty Attack

This should be explained to the patients, urate lowering frequently induces mobilisation of persisting urate crystals, resulting in the occurrence of acute flares when urate lowering drugs are started. The daily administration of 0.5-1.0 mg colchicine avoids in most cases such urate lowering drug induced attacks of inflammation [16]. Prophylaxis is recommended during the first 6 months [16]. Colchicine therapy should be maintained until their complete dissolution of crystals in joints. After prolonged successful SUA-lowering therapy gouty attacks became less frequent [16]; this may be related to the decrease in the concentration of MSU crystals in joints as a result of the SUA-lowering therapy, seen at 3 months after its initiation [16]. A minority of patients usually with long-standing poorly treated gout have attacks when starting SUA-lowering drugs even if given prophylaxis with a proper dose of colchicine. These patients in addition to SUA-lowering treatment such as allopurinol given in 100 mg increments, a more complete prophylaxis including colchicine and a small dose of an NSAID should be given. Occasionally, patients need the addition of prednisone 5 – 7.5 mg/day to colchicine for 1 – 3 months to allow introduction of SUA-lowering treatment. In difficult prophylaxis, IL-1 blocking by canakinumab or anacinra may be considered.

Correction of Hyperuricaemia by Drug Therapy

The main goal of SUA-lowering therapy is to maintain urate concentration below the saturation point for MSU. This treatment dissolves crystal deposits and cures gout while it is maintained. EULAR and ACR guidelines recommend that plasma or serum urate should be maintained at a concentration of < 6 mg/dL (360 umol/L) [16 - 18]. However this target serum level can be lowered < 5 mg/dL (300 umol/L) in the presence of severe tophaceus gout [16 - 18]. Lower SUA levels result in faster reduction of the size of tophi [16 - 18]. In patients with chronic gout, the time of disappearance of MSU crystals from signal joints induced by normalisation of SUA levels has been shown to be longer [19].

All SUA-lowering drugs, should not be started until the gouty attack has fully resolved. The urate lowering therapy could be started during an acute attack provided that the anti-inflammatory therapy has been introduced. The dose of drug used in urate lowering therapy should be low and increased until the target serum urate level is achieved. It is important to monitor SUA levels during urate lowering therapy titration, approximately every 2-4 weeks.

Three classes of drugs are approved for urate lowering therapy:xanthine oxidase inhibitors, uricosuric agents and uricase agents. Xanthine oxidase inhibitors block the synthesis of uric acid.

Drugs used to correct hyperuricaemia act either by promoting the renal excretion of urate (uricosuric agents) or by decreasing urate production by inhibiting xanthine oxidase (allopurinol and febuxostat).

Uricosuric Agents

A uricosuric agent is one that lowers the serum urate concentration by increasing the excretion of uric acid by the kidney. Uricosuric drugs aid urate excretion by the kidney with an increase in the urate clearance and the fractional excretion of filtrated urate.

Especially Useful in Urate Underexcretion

PROBENECID – 0.5-1.5 daily.

BENZBROMARONE – 50-100 mg/daily.

LESINURAD – 200 mg/daily.

Uricosuric drugs are recommended to correct hyperuricaemia when there is defective renal excretion of urate. These drugs are contraindicated if a past medical history indicated renal calculi or poor urine volume (<1 ml/min). They are ineffective in the presence of renal disease with a glomerular filtration rate (GFR) of less than 60 ml/min.

Mechanism of Action of LESINURAT (ZURAMPIC)

Lesinurad reduces serum acid levels by inhibiting the function of transporter proteins involved in uric acid reabsorption in the kidney. Lesinurad inhibited the function of two apical transporters responsible for uric reabsorption, uric acid transporter 1 (URAT1) and organic anion transporter 4 (OAT4). URAT1 is responsible for the majority of the reabsorption of filtered uric acid from the renal tubular lumen.

Zurampic in dose 200 mg in the morning is indicated in combination with a xanthine oxidase inhibitor for the treatment of hyperuricaemia associated with gout in patients who have not achieved target serum acid levels with a xanthine oxidase inhibitor alone.

Zurampic is not recommended for the treatment of asymptomatic hyperuricaemia.

Zurampic should not be used as monotherapy.

Xanthine Oxidase Inhibiting Drugs

Allopurinol

Allopurinol is become the main urate-lowering drug and now it is used as first-line urate-lowering therapy.

Allopurinol is useful in patients with urate overproduction, both primary and secondary. It reduces urate production by inhibiting xanthine oxidase.

Indication for allopurinol when an antihyperuricemic agent is required:

- Urate overproduction, primary or secondary.

- Acute uric acid nephropathy – tumor lysis syndrome.

- Nephrolithiasis of any type.

- Renal impairment (dose 100 mg/day per 30 ml/min glomerular filtration rate).

- Low urine volume.

- 24 hour urinary acid >0.42 g (2.5 mmol) (an arbitrary value on a low purine diet).

- Intolerance or allergy to uricosuric agents.

Allopurinol is a purine analogue which competitively inhibits xanthine oxidase, the enzyme responsible for the degradation of hypoxanthine and xanthine to uric acid, reducing the total amount of uric acid formed.

Allopurinol dose adjustement according to renal function is recommended by EULAR guidelines, to avoid toxicity. Azathioprine also allows to reduce dose of allopurinol to ¼, or change to Mycofenolan mofetil (MMF) [16].

The starting dose of allopurinol should be no greater than 100 mg/day, according to EULAR and ACR guidelines [18] and should be increased until a target uric acid concentration or maximum dose is achieved. Cutaneous intolerance to allopurinol occurs early in the first 3 months of allopurinol induction or dose increase and further allopurinol use should be discontinued. In patients with healthy renal function, daily doses can be raised to 300-600 mg, and even to 900 mg/day in rare cases.

The allopurinol dose needs correction according to renal function, since levels of oxypurinol, the main metabolite of allopurinol are related to the glomerular filtration rate [20]. Adaptation of the allopurinol dose can be based on the Cr clearance or the estimation of the glomerular filtration by the Cockcroft-Gault equation [20].

Azathioprine is metabolized also by xanthine oxidase; allopurinol interferes in its metabolism and their co-administration results in higher levels of azathioprine, easily leading to toxicity if the azathioprine dose is not changed. In kidney transplant recipient with gouty arthritis, mycofenolate mofetil may be substituted for azathioprine [21], allowing a safer use of xanthine oxidase inhibitors.

The allopurinol hypersensitivity syndrome remains a serious effect, which can develop within the first 3 months of allopurinol introduction [20]. Severe allopurinol-induced toxic effects arise in <1% of patients but can be life threatening, with a mortality rate of about 20% [1].

Febuxostat

Febuxostat is a non-purine selective inhibitor of xanthine oxidase indicated for the chronic management of hyperuricaemia in patients with gout. Febuxostat is not recommended for the treatment of asymptomatic hyperuricaemia.

Febuxostat has similar action to allopurinol. It has hepatic metabolism. The main advantage of febuxostat is that it is metabolized by the liver, *via* glucuronide formation and oxidation, with about 50% of the drug excreted in the stool and 50% in urine, therefore it requires no dose adjustment in patients with renal impairment.

Febuxostat 40-80-120 mg/day is used in patients who do not tolerate allopurinol and with renal insufficiency (creatinine clearance >30 ml/min) and in patients with nephrolithiasis.

Febuxostat is not recommended for patients with severe heart disease.

Allopurinol and febuxostat are contraindicated in patients who are treated with azathioprine and 6-mercaptopurine. An increase of gout flares is observed during initiation of anti-hyperuremic agents, including febuxostat. Prophylactic therapy (*i.e.* – NSAIDs or colchicines) upon initiation of treatment may be beneficial for up to six months. Adverse reaction are liver function abnormalities, nausea, arthralgia and rash.

In cases of failure of treatment with XO inhibitors alone, a combination with an uricosuric (Probenecid, Benzbromaron, Lesinurad), Losartan, Clofibrat, vitamin

C, or uricase (Rasburicase, Pegloticase) may be used.

Uricases

Uricases such as pegloticase should be used for refractory tophaceous gout. Pegloticase is a pegylated mammalian (porcine-like) recombinant uricase, at a dosage of 8 mg intravenously every 2 weeks for the treatment of severe tophaceous gout. Hydrocortisone 200 mg intravenously before infusion, may be used for infusion reaction prophylaxis.

2016 EULAR Recommendartions for the Management of Gout [16]

Overarching Principles

A. Every person with gout should be fully informed about the pathophysiology of the disease, the existence of effective treatment, associated comorbidities and the principles of managing acute attacks and eliminating urate crystals through lifelong lowering of serum uric acid (SUA) level below a target level.

B. Every person with gout should receive advice regarding lifestyle: weight loss if appropriate and avoidance of alcohol (especially beer and spirits) and sugar-sweetened drinks, heavy meals and excessive intake of meat and seafood. Low-fat dairy products should be encouraged. Regular exercise should be advised.

C. Every person with gout should be systematically screened for associated comorbidities and cardiovascular risk factors, including renal impairment, coronary heart disease, heart failure, stroke, peripheral arterial disease, obesity, hiperlipidaemia, hypertension, diabetes and smoking, which should be addressed as an integral part of the management of gout.

Final Set of 15 Recommendations

1. Acute flares of gout should be treated as early as possible. Fully informed patients should be educated to self-medicate at the first warning symptoms. The choice of drug(s) should be based on the presence of contraindications, the patuient's previous experience with treatments, time of initiation after flare onset and the number and type of joint(s) involved.

2. Recommended first-line options for acute flares are colchicines (within 12 hours of flare onset) at a loading dose of 1 mg followed 1 hour later by 0.5 mg on day 1 and/or an NSAID (plus proton pump inhibitors if appropriate), oral corticosteroid (30 – 35 mg/day of equivalent prednisolone for 3 – 5 days) or articular aspiration and injection of corticosteroids. Colchicine and NSAIDs should be avoided in patients with severe renal impairment.

3. Colchicine should not be given to patients receiving strong P-glycoprotein and/or CYPA4 inhibitors such as ciclosporin or clarythromycin.

4. In patients with frequent flares and contraindications to colchicines, NSAIDs and corticosteroid (oral and injectable), IL-1 blockers should be considered for treating flares. Current infection is considered for treating flares. Current infection is contraindication to the use of IL-1 blockers. Urate-lowering therapy (ULT) should be adjusted to achieve the hyperuricaemia target following an IL-1 blocker treatment for flare.

5. Prophylaxis against flares ahould be fully explained and discussed with the patient. Prophylaxis is recommended during the first 6 months of ULT. Recommended prophylactic treatment is colchicines, 0.5–1 mg/day a dose that should be reduced in patients with renal impairment. In cases or renal impairment or statin treatment, patients and physicians should be aware of potential neurotoxicity and/or muscular toxicity with prophylactic colchicines.

6. Co-prescription of colchicines with strong P-glycoprotein and/or CYP3A4 inhibitors should be avoided. If colchicines is not tolerated or is contraindicated, prophylaxis with NSAIDs at low dosage, if not contraindicated, should be considered.

7. Urate-lowering therapy (ULT) should be considered and discussed with every patient with a definite diagnosis of gout from the first presentation. ULT is indicated in all patients with recurrent flares, tophi, urate arthropathy and/or renal stones. Initiation of ULT is recommended close to the time of first diagnosis in patients presenting at a young age (<40 years) or with a very high SUA level (>8.0 mg/dL; 480 umol/L) and/or comorbidities (renal impairment, hypertention, ischemic heart disease, heart failure).

8. Patient with gout should receive full information and be fully involved in decision-making concerning the use of ULT.

9. For patients on ULT, serum uric acid level should be monitored and maintained to <6 mg/dl (360 umol/L) to facilitate faster dissolution of crystals is recommended for patients with severe gout (tophi, chronic arthropathy, frequent attacks) until total crystal dissolution and resolution of gout. SUA level <3 mg/dL is not recommended in the long term.

10. All ULTs should be started at a low dose and then titrated upwards until the SUA target is reached. SUA < 6 mg/dL (360 umol/L) should be maintained lifelong.

11. In patients with normal kidney function, allopurinol is recommended for first-line ULT, starting at a low dose (100 mg/day) and increasing by 100 mg increments every 2-4 weeks if required, to reach the hyperuricaemia target.

12. If the SUA target cannot be reached by an appropriate dose of allopurinol, allopurinol should be switched to febuxostat or a uricosuric or combined with a uricosuric. Febuxostat or a uricosuric are also indicated if allopurinol cannot be tolerated.

13. In patients with renal impairment, the allopurinol maximum dosage should be adjusted to creatinine clearance. If the SUA target cannot be acxhieved at this dose, the patient should be switched to febuxostat or given benzbromarone with or without allopurinol, except in patients with estimated glomerular filtration rate <30 mL/min.

14. In patients with crystal-proven, severe debilitating chronic tophaceous gout and poor quality of life, in whom the SUA target cannot be reached with any other available drug at the maximal dosage (including combinations), pegloticase is indicated.

15. When gout occurs in patients receiving loop or thiazide diuretics, substitute the diuretic if possible: for hypertension consider losartan or calcium channel blockers; for hyperlipidaemia, consider a statin or fenofibrate.

REFERENCES

[1]   Bardin T, Richette P. Definition of hyperuricemia and gouty conditions. Curr Opin Rheumatol 2014; 26(2): 186-91.
        [http://dx.doi.org/10.1097/BOR.0000000000000028] [PMID: 24419750]

[2]   Roddy E, Doherty M. Epidemiology of gout. Arthritis Res Ther 2010; 12(6): 223-38.
        [http://dx.doi.org/10.1186/ar3199] [PMID: 21205285]

[3]   Krishnan E, Baker JF, Furst DE, Schumacher HR. Gout and the risk of acute myocardial infarction. Arthritis Rheum 2006; 54(8): 2688-96.
        [http://dx.doi.org/10.1002/art.22014] [PMID: 16871533]

[4]   Richette P, Bardin T. Gout. Lancet 2010; 375(9711): 318-28.
        [http://dx.doi.org/10.1016/S0140-6736(09)60883-7] [PMID: 19692116]

[5]   Martinon F, Pétrilli V, Mayor A, Tardivel A, Tschopp J. Gout-associated uric acid crystals activate the NALP3 inflammasome. Nature 2006; 440(7081): 237-41.
        [http://dx.doi.org/10.1038/nature04516] [PMID: 16407889]

[6]   Shi Y, Mucsi AD, Ng G. Monosodium urate crystals in inflammation and immunity. Immunol Rev 2010; 233(1): 203-17.
        [http://dx.doi.org/10.1111/j.0105-2896.2009.00851.x] [PMID: 20193001]

[7]   Suresh E. Diagnosis and management of gout: a rational approach. Postgrad Med J 2005; 81(959): 572-9.
        [http://dx.doi.org/10.1136/pgmj.2004.030692] [PMID: 16143687]

[8]   Zhang W, Doherty M, Pascual E, *et al.* EULAR evidence based recommendations for gout. Part I: Diagnosis. Report of a task force of the Standing Committee for International Clinical Studies Including Therapeutics (ESCISIT). Ann Rheum Dis 2006; 65(10): 1301-11.
[http://dx.doi.org/10.1136/ard.2006.055251] [PMID: 16707533]

[9]   Canoso JJ, Yood RA. Reaction of superficial bursae in response to specific disease stimuli. Arthritis Rheum 1979; 22(12): 1361-4.
[http://dx.doi.org/10.1002/art.1780221207] [PMID: 518717]

[10]   Williamson SC, Roger DJ, Petrera P, Glockner F. Acute gouty arthropathy after total knee arthroplasty. A case report. J Bone Joint Surg Am 1994; 76(1): 126-8.
[http://dx.doi.org/10.2106/00004623-199401000-00018] [PMID: 8288656]

[11]   Hahnel J, Ramaswamy R, Grainer A, *et al.* Gout. Arthroplasty following hip arthroplasty. Geriatr Orthop Surg Rehabil 2010; 1: 36-7.
[http://dx.doi.org/10.1177/2151458510373745] [PMID: 23569660]

[12]   Zhang W, Doherty M, Bardin T, *et al.* EULAR evidence based recommendationns for gout – Part II: Management report of a task force of the EULAR Standing Commottee for International Clinical Studies Including Therapeutics (ESCISIT). Ann Rheum Dis 2006; 25: 1301-11.
[http://dx.doi.org/10.1136/ard.2006.055251] [PMID: 16707533]

[13]   Grassi W, Meenagh G, Pascual E, Filippucci E. "Crystal clear"-sonographic assessment of gout and calcium pyrophosphate deposition disease. Semin Arthritis Rheum 2006; 36(3): 197-202.
[http://dx.doi.org/10.1016/j.semarthrit.2006.08.001] [PMID: 17011611]

[14]   Lumbreras B, Pascual E, Frasquet J, González-Salinas J, Rodríguez E, Hernández-Aguado I. Analysis for crystals in synovial fluid: training of the analysts results in high consistency. Ann Rheum Dis 2005; 64(4): 612-5.
[http://dx.doi.org/10.1136/ard.2004.027268] [PMID: 15769916]

[15]   Neogi T, Jansen TLThA, Dalbeth N, *et al.* 2015 Gout classification criteria: an American College of Rheumatology/European League Against Rheumatism collaborative initiative. Ann Rheum Dis 2015; 74(10): 1789-98.
[http://dx.doi.org/10.1136/annrheumdis-2015-208237] [PMID: 26359487]

[16]   Richette P, Doherty M, Pascual E, *et al.* 2016 updated EULAR evidence-based recommendations for the management of gout. Ann Rheum Dis 2017; 76(1): 29-42.
[http://dx.doi.org/10.1136/annrheumdis-2016-209707] [PMID: 27457514]

[17]   Khanna D, Fitzgerald JD, Khanna PP, *et al.* 2012 American College of Rheumatology guidelines for management of gout. Part 1: systematic nonpharmacologic and pharmacologic therapeutic approaches to hyperuricemia. Arthritis Care Res (Hoboken) 2012; 64(10): 1431-46.
[http://dx.doi.org/10.1002/acr.21772] [PMID: 23024028]

[18]   Khanna D, Khanna PP, Fitzgerald JD, *et al.* 2012 American College of Rheumatology guidelines for management of gout. Part 2: therapy and antiinflammatory prophylaxis of acute gouty arthritis. Arthritis Care Res (Hoboken) 2012; 64(10): 1447-61.
[http://dx.doi.org/10.1002/acr.21773] [PMID: 23024029]

[19]   Perez-Ruiz F, Lioté F. Lowering serum uric acid levels: what is the optimal target for improving clinical outcomes in gout? Arthritis Rheum 2007; 57(7): 1324-8.
[http://dx.doi.org/10.1002/art.23007] [PMID: 17907217]

[20]   Stamp LK, Taylor WJ, Jones PB, *et al.* Starting dose is a risk factor for allopurinol hypersensitivity syndrome: a proposed safe starting dose of allopurinol. Arthritis Rheum 2012; 64(8): 2529-36.
[http://dx.doi.org/10.1002/art.34488] [PMID: 22488501]

[21]   Gonwa T, Johnson C, Ahsan N, *et al.* Randomized trial of tacrolimus + mycophenolate mofetil or azathioprine versus cyclosporine + mycophenolate mofetil after cadaveric kidney transplantation: results at three years. Transplantation 2003; 75(12): 2048-53.
[http://dx.doi.org/10.1097/01.TP.0000069831.76067.22] [PMID: 12829910]

CHAPTER 10

Osteoarthritis

Abstract: Osteoarthritis (OA) is the most common type of arthritis. OA is the destruction of articular cartilage, subchondral bone, ligaments, joint capsules and periarticular tissues, sensory nerve endings, menisci leading to damage of the joint, limitation of motion and pain. Obesity, occupational trauma and muscle weakness are important biomechanical risk factors. Cartilage breakdown products increase synovial inflammation.

OA mainly affects the elderly. Prevalence of osteoarthritis: 80% of patients over 55 years of age have radiographic evidence of osteoarthritis. OA is the result of active biochemical, biomechanical and cellular processes.

OA is characterized by damage of the articular cartilage, osteophyte formation at the joint margins, subchondral bone sclerosis, and synovial and joint capsule thickening. These changes lead to joint degeneration and symptoms such as pain, tenderness, stiffness, loss of function and disability.

OA develops mainly in the cervical and lumbar spine joints, hips, knees, first MTP, PIP, DIP.

Risk factors of osteoarthritis are age, major joint trauma, repetitive stress and joint overload, obesity, congenital/development defects, prior inflammatory joint disease, metabolic changes and endocrine changes.

Obesity is the main modifiable risk factor for OA.

Pain or stiffness in and around one or more joints is the most common symptoms of OA.

Radiological changes are narrowing of the joint space, subchondral bone sclerosis, bone cysts, osteophytes.

Treatment OA include patient education, reduction of pain, optimization of treatment and modification of the degenerative process. First we use non-pharmacological methods, next topical capsaicin and topical NSAIDs, than acetaminophen, oral NSAIDs and finally arthroplasty.

Keywords: Acetaminophen, Arthroplasty, Articular cartilage, Bone cysts, Cervical spine, DIP, Disability, First MTP, Hips, Joint capsules, Knees, Ligaments, Limitation of motion, Loss of function, Lumbar spine joints, Menisci,

Narrowing of the joint space, Obesity, Occupational trauma, Oral NSAIDs, Osteoarthritis (OA), Osteophyte, Pain, Pain, Periarticular tissues, PIP, Sensory nerve endings, Stiffness, Subchondral bone, Subchondral bone sclerosis, Subchondral bone sclerosis, Synovial inflammation, Tenderness, Topical capsaicin, Topical NSAIDs.

INTRODUCTION

Osteoarthritis (OA) is the destruction of articular cartilage, subchondral bone, ligaments, joint capsules and periarticular tissues, sensory nerve endings, and menisci, leading to damage of the joint, limitation of motion and pain. These changes may be accompanied by synovitis caused by the breakdown products of cartilage and bone. Osteoarthritis is the most common type of arthritis. Obesity, occupational trauma and muscle weakness are important biomechanical risk factors which determine the site and severity of the disease.

Prevalence of osteoarthritis: 60% of patients over 35 years of age have arthralgia. 80% of patients over 55 years of age have radiographic evidence of osteoarthritis. Only 5% of patients between 15-44 years have osteoarthritis, as well as 30% of patients between 45-65 years and 60% of patients between 65-75 years [1]. OA mainly affects the elderly but should not be considered a simple consequence of aging. OA is not considered as a "degenerative" or "tear and wear" disease but the result of active biochemical, biomechanical and cellular processes.

In 2010 OA was identified as one of the top cause of disability in the future [1]. OA affects an increasing amount of people, due to the obesity and aging of the population.

Joints in humans were formed when our ancestors moved on four legs so OA develops in the joints, whose function has changed: the cervical and lumbar spine joints, hips, knees, first MTP, PIP, DIP.

Cartilage is composed of type II collagen, proteoglycans and glycoproteins, which are degraded in OA by activated proteases (matrix metalloproteinases [MMP], tissue plasminogen activator [t-PA], plasmin, cathepsins and aggrecanases). Articular cartilage (a subset of hyaline cartilage) is composed of extracellular matrix, which contains collagen (type II fibrils with both collagen IX and XI) and proteoglycans. Among the proteoglycans, aggrecan is a central core protein bearing numerous glycosaminoglycan chains of chondroitin sulphate, which are attached to hyaluronic acid. The molecular complexes are able to retain water. Along with type II collagen, aggrecan forms a major structural component of articular cartilage gives the cartilage its functional properties, such as compressibility and elasticity.

Chondrocytes are the cells in the extracelluar matrix that are responsible for the production, maintenance and destruction of the cartilaginous matrix. Chondrocytes have low metabolic activity and can survive under hypoxic conditions. Nutrients come from the synovial fluid and from subchondral bone, maintaining its cellular activities. The chondrocyte itself possesses little regenerative properties.

OA is a disease of the joints, involving different structures and influencing their functional interaction.

PATHOLOGY OF OA

OA is characterized by damage of the articular cartilage, osteophyte formation at the joint margins, subchondral bone sclerosis, and synovial and joint capsule thickening. These changes lead to joint degeneration and symptoms such as pain, tenderness, stiffness, loss of function and disability.

The main macroscopic changes in an osteoarthritic joint are: 1 - reduced joint space related to loss of articular cartilage; 2 - subchondral bone with hypertrophic reaction (sclerosis) and new bone formation (osteophytes) at the joint margins; 3 - inflammation and hyperplasia of the synovial membrane and joint capsule.

In physiological conditions, the water-rich articular cartilage forms a soft cap on top of the bones, allowing smooth movement and transition. In the first stages of the disease, before clinical signs and symptoms start to develop, the smooth surface of the articular cartilage becomes roughened with small irregularities and superficial clefts. During the disease, the cracks become deeper, lesions may grow and connect, thereby increasing the damaged surface. Clefts become focal erosions and ulcerations, ultimately exposing parts of the underlying bone. Changes in the subchondral bone show sclerosis or thickening and due to loss of cartilage. Osteophytes (bony outgrowths) are formed at the joint margins. The formation of subchondral cysts and areas of bone marrow oedema may also occur.

Chondrocytes release matrix-degrading enzymes and inflammatory cytokines that contribute to the progressive destruction. Another feature of OA is chondrocyte cell death, which occurs through apoptosis and necrosis.

In the early stages of disease, water content is increasing, leading to tissue oedema and weakening of the collagen network. Type II collagen synthesis decreases and is replaced to some extent by type I collagen. Proteoglycan content strongly decreases and shorter glycosaminoglycans appear. The concentration of type 6 keratan sulfate increases during the osteoarthritic process to the detriment of type 4 keratan sulfate. These changes alter the ability of the extracellular matrix to retain water, changing the distribution of force in the weight-bearing zone and the transmission of load to the subchondral bone. The loss of proteoglycans may be partially reversible, but it changes the properties of the extracellular matrix, making the collagen structure more susceptible to degradation by collagenases.

In OA there is an imbalance between synthesis components of articular cartilage and their degradation by tissue inhibitors of metalloproteinases [TIMP], α2 macroglobulin and plasminogen activator inhibitor [PAI-1]. IL-1 and TNFα stimulates the synthesis of nitric oxide and cartilage-degrading enzymes.

Repair is made by IGF-1 and TGFβ, which stimulate the biosynthesis of proteoglycans and collagen and reduce the number of IL-1 receptors on chondrocytes. The most important factor stimulating the production of proteoglycan is repeated joint load as regular movements are necessary for their normal function. Blocking the enzyme or a cytokine involved in joint destruction or stimulation of synthesis of articular cartilage components is not enough to stop the disease.

In OA, the association between matrix-degrading enzymes (including matrix metalloproteinases (MMPs) and aggrecanases) and cartilage damage has been observed [2]. ADAMTS (a disintegrin and metalloproteinase with thrombospondin motifs) are matrix degrading enzymes, and a family of peptidases. Aggrecanase 1 (or ADAMTS-4) and aggrecanase 2 (or ADAMTS-5 which is the same as ADAMTS-11) play an important role in the breakdown of aggrecan [3].

OA chondrocytes produce matrix-degrading enzymes including MMP-1, MMP-3, MMP-9, MMP-13, MMP-14 and aggrecanases ADAMTS-4 and ADAMTS-5, therefore cartilage cells may degrade of their own tissue [4]. The activity of MMPs is regulated by serine proteases (plasminogen activator, plasminogen, plasmin), free radicals, cathepsin and some-membrane-type MMPs. Their effect is also controlled by inhibitors including the tissue inhibitors of metalloproteinases (TIMPs) by stoichiometric inhibition and the inhibitor of plasminogen activator. Therefore, the balance between the amounts of MMPs and TIMPs in the cartilage determines the level of degradation [4].

Breakdown of type II collagen is due to collagenase-1 (MMP-1) and collagenase-3 (MMP-13). Their expression differs proteolytic potency, target sensitivity, expression and localisation.

Stromelysin-1 (MMP-3), Stromelysin-2 (MMP-10) and Stromelysin-3 (MMP-11) are also involved in the degradation of cartilage.

The transforming growth factor-ß (TGFß) family, bone morphogenetic proteins (BMPs) and the Wnt signalling cascade are involved in the pathogenesis of OA. TGF ß is considered an anabolic factor for cartilage. It has a physiological role in healthy cartilage, however the pathway and its downstream effects is dysregulated in OA [5].

BMPs have chondroprotective and stimulating properties however may lead to further differentiation of chondrocytes (hypertrophy) and stimulate osteophyte formation [6].

Activation and suppression of the Wnt-b-catenin cascade lead to OA in rodent models. Wnts have a role in the terminal differentiation of chondrocytes. The balanced control of Wnt signalling in articular cartilage is needed for joint homeostasis.

Cartilage breakdown products increase synovial inflammation. The inflamed synovium produces catabolic and proinflammatory mediators that lead to excess production of proteolytic enzymes responsible for cartilage breakdown, creating a positive feedback loop. The most common feature of inflammation of synovial tissue is hyperplasia, with an increased number of lining cells and a mixed cellular infiltrate [7]. Macrophages and T cells are the most common cells in OA synovial tissue [8]. Inflammatory cells and their cytokines are present in both early and late OA [9].

Different triggers of the innate immune system may be already active early in the disease process in OA. These triggers include matrix molecules, complement and crystals.

IL1ß and TNFα are important cytokines for the cartilage catabolic process [10]. IL-1 is synthesised in concentrations that are capable of inducing the expression of MMP and other catabolic genes. IL-1 is localised with TNFα, MMP-1, MMP-3, MMP-8, MMP-13 and type II collagen cleavage epitopes in OA cartilage. IL-1 induce ADAMTS-4 and TNFα induces both ADAMTS-4 and ADAMTS-5. Both IL-1 and TNFα increase the synthesis of prostaglandin E2 (PGE2) by stimulating the gene expression and the activity of COX-2, microsomal PGE synthetase-1 (mPGES-1) and soluble phospholipase A2 (sPLA2). They also increase the amount of nitric oxide *via* inducible nitric oxide synthetase (iNOS or NOS2) and induce production of other cytokines, such as the proinflammatory cytokines IL-6, LIF (leucocyte inhibiting factor), IL-17 and IL-18 and chemokines such as IL-8. IL-1 and TNFα suppress a number of genes associated with the differentiated chondrocyte phenotype, including *aggrecan (AGAN)* and *type II collagen (COL2A1)* [11].

Chondrocytes bear oestrogen receptors and their stimulation can trigger the production of growth factors. The concentration of oestrogens decreases during menopause, leading to a decrease in the synthesis of these growth factors. It has been shown that adipokines (resistin, leptin and adiponectin) are found in synovial fluid [12] and have multiple functions. Obesity-related OA can affect both the weight-bearing joints and also the hands, suggesting a role for the adipose tissue and systemic adipokines [13].

Etiopathogenesis of Osteoarthritis

Genetics factors for 50% to 60% of OA, and obesity is another risk factor. Joint injury increases the risk five-fold. Jobs that require kneeling or squatting such as farming also increase the risk.

Risk Factors of Osteoarthritis: Age, major joint trauma, repetitive stress and joint overload, obesity, congenital/development defects, prior inflammatory joint disease, metabolic changes and endocrine changes.

Obesity is the main modifiable risk factor for OA. The link between obesity and OA is stronger in women than in men.

Other metabolic disorders, such as hyperglycaemia, have been associated with OA occurrence and severity [14]. Diabetes was associated with a risk for bilateral knee OA and hypercholesterolemia was independently associated with generalized OA [15].

Patients age is the best recognized risk factor, because the incidence of radiographic and symptomatic OA increases with age. The frequency of hip OA increases at about the same rate in women and men.

Sex hormones seem to be involved in OA pathogenesis since the prevalence of OA is higher in women than in men, especially during menopause. This can be explained by the presence of oestrogen receptors in chondrocytes and modulation of their function depending on sex hormones.

The occurrence of OA is associated with physical activity during work like climbing of stairs, farming, prolonged standing, weight lifting and walking over rough ground.

Carpo-metacarpal OA of the thumb is associated with tailoring and dressmaking, while severe OA of the right thumb, index and middle fingers occurs in dentists [16].

Joint deformity is associated with OA. Congenital abnormal joint shapes, such as acetabular dysplasia, slipped capital femoral epiphysis, abnormal femoral head shape or abnormal femoral neck shaft angle of the hip may be etiologies of secondary OA. Limb fractures may cause of secondary OA.

Meniscus damage has an important role in OA pathophysiology [17]. Meniscectomy increases the risk of knee OA twofold and more if it is combined with ligament injury.

Walking in high-heeled shoes is a risk for developing degenerative changes in the patellofemoral and medial compartment of the knee [18].

The most important risk factors for OA are "non-modifiable", including female gender, joint malformation and previous trauma.

Genetic factors also contribute to OA [19]. Genome-wide association studies (GWAS) and meta-analyses on large datasets and multiple cohorts identified regions with multiple candidate genes [20]. Recent genetic studies in primary OA, two pathways may be involved in OA aetiology.

The first pathway is the inflammatory pathway: variants in the *IL1* gene cluster, the *HLA* cluster and the *cyclooxygenase 2 (COX2)* gene [21]. Association with the *IL1* gene cluster are shown for knee, hip and hand OA [22].

The second pathway is involved in early skeletal development processes or maintenance of cartilage and bone: *growth/differentiation factor 5 (GDF5)* [23], *frizzled-related protein β (FRZB)* [24], *transforming growth factor (TGF) β1 SMAD3* [25] *and type 2 iodothyronine deiodinase (DIO2)* [26].

The strongest genetic signal is the *GDF5* gene and is also known as cartilage derived morphogenic protein 1 (CDMP1). *GDF5* stimulates proliferation and differentiation of chondrocytes. Lack of or a reduction in *GDF5* may result in abnormal ligament laxity and contributes to OA development through joint instability [27]. *GDF5* also contributes to subchondral bone modeling and remodeling with reduced *GDF5* levels associated with abnormal structure of the collagen network [27].

Epigenetic regulation is DNA methylation, as de-methylation leads to an increase in the gene transcription. Enzymes involved in cartilage breakdown in OA undergo epigenetic regulation (*MMP-3, MMP-9, MMP-13, ADAMTS-4*) and *IL1B* promoter region in chondrocytes and leptin which regulates expression of *MMP-13* [28]. Growth factors and proinflammatory cytokines regulate the methylation state of pro-degradative agent genes.

Clinical Features: tenderness, joint swelling, crepitus, limitation of motion, deformity, instability.

Pain or stiffness in and around one or more joints is the most common symptoms of OA. Imaging helps in the diagnosis.

Pain is the first symptom of OA. It occurs after joint use and is relieved by rest. With disease progression, pain occurs with minimal activity or even at rest and finally during sleep. OA pain is not usually present at night or at rest, however there are exceptions: patients with mild OA using joints for several hours, especially during sport; patients with advanced OA and destructive arthropathy; and patients with an acute inflammatory flare of OA mimicking inflammatory arthropathy, especially regarding erosive hand OA. Cartilage has no nerve supply and is insensitive to pain. The pain in OA arises from non-cartilaginous structures such as periostium, intra-articular ligaments, pressure on subchondral bone with venous engorgement, intramedullary engorgement, capsular distension, and alterations in synovium or tendons and fascia. Pain may be from associated bursitis or periarticular tissue such as tendons and fascia.

Stiffness occurs in the morning or after inactivity during the day. Morning stiffness resolves after around 15 min or less.

Limitations of motion and function develop as OA progresses and are related to joint surface changes with reduced joint space, muscle spasm or decreased strength leading to instability and mechanical block from osteophytes and loose bodies. Joint prioprioceptor activity may be changed. Everyday activities such as kneeling for knee, climbing stairs, walking and performing house-hold chores are difficult to perform. Impaired hand function is associated with the severity of OA, pain, joint involvement and the presence of nodes [29].

Physical examination confirms and characterizes joint involvement and excludes pain and functional syndromes arising from other causes, including peri-articular structures, neurological disorders and inflammatory arthritis. A normal examination does not rule out the diagnosis of OA.

The symptoms such as joint swelling – joint enlargement results from joint effusion or osteophytes or synovitis. A synovial effusion may be seen during OA flares, but can also occur during chronic phases.

Joint tenderness: joints are tender during active motion testing and under pressure. Limited passive movement can be the first and only physical sign of symptomatic OA. Crepitus is felt on passive or active mobilisationn of an OA joint and may result from cartilage loss, joint surface irregularity or intra-articular debris. Although crepitus can be present with passive motion, it is most commonly demonstrated by active motion of the joint.

Joint deformities and subluxation represent advanced disease due to cartilage loss, collapse of subchondral bone, formation of bone cysts and bony overgrowth.

IMAGING OA

Radiological examination is not necessary to confirm the diagnosis of hand, knee or forefoot OA. Some regions and clinical symptoms need a radiological examination to support the history and clinical assessment and to aid in the exclusion of other diseases including avascular osteonecrosis, Paget's disease. algodystrophy, inflammatory arthropathies and stress fractures.

Radiological Changes: narrowing of the joint space, subchondral bone sclerosis, bone erosions, osteophytes, bone cysts.

Weight-bearing X-rays are mandatory for knee and hip OA.

Clinical symptoms and radiographic findings are poorly correlated, many joints with radiographic evidence of OA remain asymptomatic and the joints of many patients with severe symptoms show minimal changes on X-ray [30].

Joint space narrowing is due to a decreased volume of articular cartilage, and also to meniscal cartilage lesions and cartilage extrusion [31].

MRI is used to exclude tumour or avascular osteonecrosis. Cartilage thickness is detected early by MRI [32]. Bone marrow oedema can be observed. Meniscus tears seen on MRI are common in middle-aged and older adults, with or without knee pain. Quantitative MRI is a non-invasive measures of cartilage degeneration in the early stages of joint degeneration [33].

Ultrasound is only useful for detecting joint effusions, including a minimal effusion undetectable upon clinical examination, changes in cartilage such as fibrillation of cartilage or cleft formation, synovitis and osteophytes. Popliteal cysts can be shown on ultrasound and compression of adjacent vascular structures. Ultrasonography is used in hand OA to differentiate between erosive and non-erosive OA. Ultrasonography can be used to perform aspirations and injections in the joint and peri-articular tissue. However, ultrasound cannot be used to visualize the entire cartilage surface due to artifacts caused by the position of the probe, and by inter- and intra-observer variations.

Arthroscopy may show cartilage, synovial membranes, osteophytes and meniscal lesions. This is used less due to the use of MRI.

Laboratory Tests

Blood tests are not indicated to confirm the diagnosis of OA. The erythrocyte sedimentation rate and C-reactive protein concentrations are within the normal range for age. Low titre of rheumatoid factor can be found. Laboratory tests may be performed to rule out a metabolic arthropathy such as gout or haemochromatosis or inflammatory arthritis.

Synovial fluid in primary OA is non-inflammatory.

CLINICAL SUBSETS OF OA

OA affects distal interphalangeal joints, proximal interphalangeal joints, the trapezio-metacarpal joint, the knee, hip and intervertebral facet joints.

Wrists, elbows, metacarpophalangeal joints and shoulders are affected less by OA, and this may suggest the presence of secondary OA or another diagnosis.

HAND JOINTS OSTEOARTHRITIS

Heberden's nodes – DIP joints and Bouchard's nodes – PIP joints.

The hand is one of the most common sites of OA. Post-menopausal women are more frequently affected than men (sex ratio =10: 1) and genetic factors explain familial aggregation [34]. Hand OA begins after 40 years of age [35] and affects multiple hand joints such as the distal interphalangeal, proximal interphalangeal and first carpometacarpal joints of the hand [36]. The four main complains of hand OA are: pain on use, mild morning stiffness, disfigurement and disability, with impaired manual skills and decreased hand mobility leading to restriction of occupational activity.

OA involves the first carpometacarpal joints, causing painful motion, tenderness, and squared deformation of the radial base of the thumb, and fixed adduction that leads to severe disability [37].

HIP JOINT OSTEOARTHRITIS

Hip pain may develop slowly and may cause a painful shuffling gait. Pain is felt on the outer aspect of the hip or in the groin area, as well as on the inner thigh, buttocks, or **knee**. Limitation of joint motion makes sitting down and rising difficult. With disease progress, limb shortening may occur.

Advanced OA presents as limited range of movement. The leg is held in external rotation with the hip flexed and adducted. Quadriceps muscle weakness is common.

KNEE JOINT OSTEOARTHRITIS

Varus Deformity of Knee Like the Letter O

Valgus deformity of knee like the letter X.

Two forms of changes: 1 - a process on the back surface of the patella causing pain while climbing stairs; 2 - meniscal damage on the proximal epiphyseal part of the tibia causing joint space narrowing, varus or valgus deformity of the knee and pain when standing up and walking.

OA can involve the medial tibiofemoral, the lateral tibiofemoral and the patellofemoral compartments. The lateral tibiofemoral compartment is involved in women with a genu-valgum misalignment. Varus and valgus angulation affects the range of motion and accelerate joint space narrowing and enhances the development of OA.

The knee can lock if loose bodies or fragment of cartilage get into the joint space. This can be distinguish between the stiffness experienced after long immobilisation of a limb and true mechanical locking, which suggests a meniscus lesion.

A popliteal (Baker's) cyst communicating with the joint space is common. The cyst may rupture into the posterior calf muscles, mimicking venous thrombosis.

The pain of patellofemoral OA is specific: pain occurs during climbing or descending stars, while pain during walking on level ground is a symptom from the tibiofemoral compartment. Involvement of the patellofemoral compartment can cause anterior or posterior pain. Patellofemoral pain is due to the patella pressing on the femoral condyles, or after patella subluxation or blocking elevation of the patella during quadriceps contraction when the knee is extended. Patellofemoral OA is better tolerated than tibiofemoral OA.

Classical features are focal joint space narrowing, osteophytes, subchondral bone sclerosis and subchondral cysts on X-rays [38].

An axis of 0° degree to 3°of varus is within normal limits [39].

Spondyloarthritis involves diarthrodial joints, intervertebral fibrocartilaginous discs and vertebral bodies in spine particularly in the cervical and lumbar regions. Osteophytes of the vertebrae can narrow the foramina and compress nerve roots producing additional back pain.

SPONDYLOARTHRITIS OF CERVICAL SPINE

Clinical features – limitation of movement of cervical spine – lateral bend and rotation. Brachial neuralgic syndrome – pain of shoulder or scapulae radiating along upper extremity – caused by compression of nerve roots of C5 – C7. Changes on the level of C2 – C4 may lead to neurologic problems and may compromise blood flow through the vertebral arteries leading to dizziness, visual problems, headaches and vertigo.

SPONDYLOARTHRITIS OF LUMBAR SPINE

Clinical features: frequency increases with age, changes are present in X-rays in 50% of patients over 50 years in both sexes, clinical symptoms are not always present. Physical examination reveals a reduction in lumbar lordosis (kyphosis and scoliosis rarely forms), limitation of movement, pain during palpation and tenderness.

MANAGEMENT: relieve lumbar spine by rest – laying in a chair-like position – 90°angle in the knees and hips, weight loss if overweight, NSAIDs, analgetic therapy, physiotherapy (interferential, diadynamic current, massages).

PROTRUSION OF THE DISC L3/L4 – compression of L4 root.

Clinical features: – back pain, which radiates to postero-lateral area of the thigh, anterior area of the shin, disturbances of superficial sensation in these areas.

PROTRUSION OF THE DISC L4/L5 – compression of L5 root.

Clinical features: pain radiating from the posterior area of the thigh through postero-lateral area of the shin to the toe. Weak patella reflex. Decreased superficial sensation on the external area of the shin and toe. Difficulties with heel walking.

PROTRUSION OF THE DISC L5/S1 – compression of S1 root.

Clinical features: pain radiating from the posterior area of the thigh and the shin to the 5th toe. Suppressed jumping reflex. Decreased superficial sensation on the external area of feet and toes 3 to 5. Difficulties with walking on toes.

Management

OA Diagnosis:

1. Joint pain (VAS scale).
2. Characteristic location of changes: knee joints, hands: DIP, PIP, spine and hip

joints.
3. Clinical assessment of movement range (scales: WOMAC, Lequesne).
4. Imaging (plain radiographs, ultrasonography, magnetic resonance imaging, computer tomography).
5. Arthroscopy.

In 2014 NICE Modified General Recommendations for the Management of Osteoarthritis [40].

The main goals of treatment include patient education, reduction of pain, optimization of treatment and modification of the degenerative process.

Current treatment of OA by NICE include:

1. Non-pharmacological methods.
2. Topical capsaicin and topical NSAIDs.
3. Acetaminophen.
4. Oral NSAIDs.
5. Arthroplasty.

Nonpharmacological methods: education and consulting, weight loss (if the patient is obese), exercise, physical therapy, spa treatment, orthopedic supplies.

Patients should exercise as a primary treatment, regardless of age, comorbidity, severity of pain and disability. Treatment must be determined individually for each patient and change in behavior in relation to exercise, weight reduction and use of appropriate shoes must be ensured. Comorbidities such as kidney disease and cardiovascular disease are a contraindication to the use of NSAIDs. Depression increases the perception of pain. Joints are constructed so that regular movements are necessary for their normal function. Aerobic exercises are the best (fitness training) because they increase activity, improve mood, sleep, reduce obesity, and have a positive effect on other diseases, eg. diabetes, heart failure and hypertension. Quadricep and gluteal muscle exercises reduce muscle tension, improve balance and reduce the risk of falls. Physical training is the primary treatment for OA.

Rehabilitation Treatment: aerobics, exercises to increase muscle strength, limb axis correction, walking sticks, crutches, orthopedic insoles, proper shoes, elastic bands, devices to facilitate daily activity.

Physiotherapy Treatment: cryotherapy, thermotherapy, diadynamic current, transcutaneous electrical nerve stimulation (TENS), laser therapy, ultrasonics, magnetotherapy and iontophoresis.

CRYOTHERAPY

Local cryotherapy or systemic cryotherapy – first used by Yamauchi in 1979. It was observed that a patient, who escaped from hospital and was found in the mountains almost frozen, was free of symptoms of rheumatic diseases, such as joint pain and swelling. Yamauchi began treating patients with temp. to –160°C in cold cabin for 2-3 min. Cryotherapy decreases joint pain and muscle tension, as well as reduces β endorphin levels.

Thermotherapy: Hydrotherapy (bath, shower), compression (*e.g.* mud), paraffin compresses, hot air or steam, infrared, ultraviolet radiation therapy, high-frequency currents.

Ultrasonic acoustic waves with frequency greater than 20 kHz, which is above the range of human hearing (16 Hz to 20 kHz). Ultrasound improves blood circulation, nerve conduction, reduces skeletal muscle tone, and has an analgetic effect.

Magnetotherapy – application of a pulsating magnetic field, which has anti-inflammatory, analgesic and sedative effects, as well as causing vasodilation and accelerates wound healing.

Diadynamic currents are composed of half-ciscular shaped and last 10 ms. They have analgesic and anti-inflammatory effects. There are 6 types of currents: DF, MF, CP, LP, RS, MM.

Laser – lasers produce a coherent and monochromatic light radiation, causing vasodilation, increasing the rate of blood flow through capillaries, increasing the partial pressure of oxygen and stimulating enzymatic processes in cells.

Pharmacological treatment of OA according to NICE [40].

Treatment should begin with topical NSAIDs and capsaicin, as there are no gastrointestinal complications. NSAIDs are administered in the form of creams, gels or spray three times a day to the skin, since many patients' pain is caused by periarticular changes and not intraarticular ones. Capsaicin is an alkaloid obtained from chili peppers, which selectively binds to the protein of TRPV1 (transient receptor potential vanilloid type 1), a heat-activated calcium channel on the peripheral surface of the type C nociceptive fibers. Prolonged activation of these neurons by repeated applications of capsaicin gradually lowers presynaptic concentration of substance P – a key neurotransmitter of pain and heat, thereby reducing conduction of painful stimuli.

In order to relieve the pain which is not responding to topical NSAIDs, paracetamol must be given at a dose from 1 g to 4 g in divided doses per day. Paracetamol inhibits COX3 and does not cause serious interactions with other drugs in the elderly, such as warfarin. If oral acetaminophen does not reduce pain, the NSAID is currently a second line drug + PPI.

Confirmed risk factors associated with NSAIDs: induced peptic ulcer complications – history of prior ulcers, GI haemorrhage, dyspepsia, and/or previous NSAIDs intolerance, age 65 and over, higher doses and toxic NSAIDs, use of GCS, anticoagulants, H2 blockers, Helicobacter pylori infection, concomitant use of more than one NSAID, female, smoking and alcohol use.

Drugs reducing muscle tension, *e.g.* Tolperisone, are also of great importance.

Intraarticular GCS administration is recommended for the same joints however not exceeding 2-3 times every 2-3 months, due to the risk of necrosis of cartilage and subchondral bone. Methylprednisolone, betamethasone, triamcinolone have an analgesic effect and improve joint function for up to several weeks.

Opioid- tramadol at a dose of 50-100 mg 2-3 times a day (only in patients with very severe pain and short duration of use). Strong opioids – fentanyl patches (Durogesic) every 72 hours. Side effects include nausea, vomiting, constipation, drowsiness, dizziness and respiratory depression.

NICE does not recommend the use of glucosamine and chondroitin preparations, administration of intraarticular hyaluronate, arthroscopic treatment (lavage or debridement) except in patients with a history of mechanical joint locking (the presence of joint loose bodies in X-ray examination is not enough) and oral NSAIDs prior to using non-pharmacological treatment and paracetamol [40].

Arthroplasty should be performed before the onset of permanent and reduced quality of life. Corrective osteotomy, synovectomy, debridement, joint arthroscopy should not be performed when the only indication is the presence of loose bodies in the joint.

In cases of disc prolapsed, causing compression of marrow or roots as well as paralysis, immediate surgery is required.

In cases where a prolapsed disc does not cause compression of marrow or roots, or paralysis, only conservative treatment is needed: NSAIDs, drugs decreasing muscle spasms, physical therapy, laying in a chair-like position – 90° angle of knee and hip joints.

Early diagnosis and early management are of key importance. Neuromuscular training – exercises designed to strengthen and increase joint stability and functioning can delay progression of the disease and improve the patient's ability to perform normal activities of daily life. Mesenchymal stem cells therapy is the promising therapy for the future.

REFERENCES

[1]   Vos T, Flaxman AD, Naghavi M, *et al.* Years lived with disability (YLDs) for 1160 sequelae of 289 diseases and injuries 1990-2010: a systematic analysis for the Global Burden of Disease Study 2010. Lancet 2012; 380(9859): 2163-96.
[http://dx.doi.org/10.1016/S0140-6736(12)61729-2] [PMID: 23245607]

[2]   Goldring MB, Goldring SR. Osteoarthritis. J Cell Physiol 2007; 213(3): 626-34.
[http://dx.doi.org/10.1002/jcp.21258] [PMID: 17786965]

[3]   Fosang AJ, Rogerson FM. Identifying the human aggrecanase. Osteoarthritis Cartilage 2010; 18(9): 1109-16.
[http://dx.doi.org/10.1016/j.joca.2010.06.014] [PMID: 20633677]

[4]   Cawston TE, Young DA. Proteinases involved in matrix turnover during cartilage and bone breakdown. Cell Tissue Res 2010; 339(1): 221-35.
[http://dx.doi.org/10.1007/s00441-009-0887-6] [PMID: 19915869]

[5]   van der Kraan PM, Goumans MJ, Blaney Davidson E, ten Dijke P. Age-dependent alteration of TGF-β signalling in osteoarthritis. Cell Tissue Res 2012; 347(1): 257-65.
[http://dx.doi.org/10.1007/s00441-011-1194-6] [PMID: 21638205]

[6]   Lories RJ, Luyten FP. The bone-cartilage unit in osteoarthritis. Nat Rev Rheumatol 2011; 7(1): 43-9.
[http://dx.doi.org/10.1038/nrrheum.2010.197] [PMID: 21135881]

[7]   de Lange-Brokaar BJ, Ioan-Facsinay A, van Osch GJ, *et al.* Synovial inflammation, immune cells and their cytokines in osteoarthritis: a review. Osteoarthritis Cartilage 2012; 20(12): 1484-99.
[http://dx.doi.org/10.1016/j.joca.2012.08.027] [PMID: 22960092]

[8]   Kennedy A, Fearon U, Veale DJ, Godson C. Macrophages in synovial inflammation. Front Immunol 2011; 2: 52-64.
[http://dx.doi.org/10.3389/fimmu.2011.00052] [PMID: 22566842]

[9]   Benito MJ, Veale DJ, FitzGerald O, van den Berg WB, Bresnihan B. Synovial tissue inflammation in early and late osteoarthritis. Ann Rheum Dis 2005; 64(9): 1263-7.
[http://dx.doi.org/10.1136/ard.2004.025270] [PMID: 15731292]

[10]   Fernandes JC, Martel-Pelletier J, Pelletier JP. The role of cytokines in osteoarthritis pathophysiology. Biorheology 2002; 39(1-2): 237-46.
[PMID: 12082286]

[11]   Goldring MB, Otero M. Inflammation in osteoarthritis. Curr Opin Rheumatol 2011; 23(5): 471-8.
[http://dx.doi.org/10.1097/BOR.0b013e328349c2b1] [PMID: 21788902]

[12]   Schäffler A, Ehling A, Neumann E, *et al.* Adipocytokines in synovial fluid. JAMA 2003; 290(13): 1709-10.
[PMID: 14519703]

[13]   Sellam J, Berenbaum F. Is osteoarthritis a metabolic disease? Joint Bone Spine 2013; 80(6): 568-73.
[http://dx.doi.org/10.1016/j.jbspin.2013.09.007] [PMID: 24176735]

[14]   Cimmino MA, Parodi M. Risk factors for osteoarthritis. Semin Arthritis Rheum 2005; 34(6) (Suppl. 2): 29-34.
[http://dx.doi.org/10.1016/j.semarthrit.2004.03.009] [PMID: 16206954]

[15]   Stürmer T, Sun Y, Sauerland S, *et al.* Serum cholesterol and osteoarthritis. The baseline examination of the Ulm Osteoarthritis Study. J Rheumatol 1998; 25(9): 1827-32.
[PMID: 9733467]

[16]   Fontana L, Neel S, Claise JM, Ughetto S, Catilina P. Osteoarthritis of the thumb carpometacarpal joint in women and occupational risk factors: a case-control study. J Hand Surg Am 2007; 32(4): 459-65. [http://dx.doi.org/10.1016/j.jhsa.2007.01.014] [PMID: 17398355]

[17]   Roemer FW, Guermazi A, Hunter DJ, *et al.* The association of meniscal damage with joint effusion in persons without radiographic osteoarthritis: the Framingham and MOST osteoarthritis studies. Osteoarthritis Cartilage 2009; 17(6): 748-53. [http://dx.doi.org/10.1016/j.joca.2008.09.013] [PMID: 19008123]

[18]   Kerrigan DC, Johansson JL, Bryant MG, Boxer JA, Della Croce U, Riley PO. Moderate-heeled shoes and knee joint torques relevant to the development and progression of knee osteoarthritis. Arch Phys Med Rehabil 2005; 86(5): 871-5. [http://dx.doi.org/10.1016/j.apmr.2004.09.018] [PMID: 15895330]

[19]   Reynard LN, Loughlin J. Insights from human genetic studies into the pathways involved in osteoarthritis. Nat Rev Rheumatol 2013; 9(10): 573-83. [http://dx.doi.org/10.1038/nrrheum.2013.121] [PMID: 23958796]

[20]   Evangelou E, Kerkhof HJ, Styrkarsdottir U, *et al.* A meta-analysis of genome-wide association studies identifies novel variants associated with osteoarthritis of the hip. Ann Rheum Dis 2014; 73(12): 2130-6. [http://dx.doi.org/10.1136/annrheumdis-2012-203114] [PMID: 23989986]

[21]   Güler VG, Yalın S, Berköz M, *et al.* The association between cyclooxygenase-2 (COX-2/PTGS2) gene polymorphism and osteoarthritis. Eklem Hastalik Cerrahisi 2011; 22(1): 22-7. [PMID: 21417982]

[22]   Attur M, Wang HY, Kraus VB, *et al.* Radiographic severity of knee osteoarthritis is conditional on *interleukin 1 receptor antagonist* gene variations. Ann Rheum Dis 2010; 69(5): 856-61. [http://dx.doi.org/10.1136/ard.2009.113043] [PMID: 19934104]

[23]   Miyamoto Y, Mabuchi A, Shi D, *et al.* A functional polymorphism in the 5' UTR of *GDF5* is associated with susceptibility to osteoarthritis. Nat Genet 2007; 39(4): 529-33. [http://dx.doi.org/10.1038/2005] [PMID: 17384641]

[24]   Evangelou E, Chapman K, Meulenbelt I, *et al.* Large-scale analysis of association between *GDF5* and *FRZB* variants and osteoarthritis of the hip, knee, and hand. Arthritis Rheum 2009; 60(6): 1710-21. [http://dx.doi.org/10.1002/art.24524] [PMID: 19479880]

[25]   Valdes AM, Spector TD, Tamm A, *et al.* Genetic variation in the *SMAD3* gene is associated with hip and knee osteoarthritis. Arthritis Rheum 2010; 62(8): 2347-52. [http://dx.doi.org/10.1002/art.27530] [PMID: 20506137]

[26]   Meulenbelt I, Min JL, Bos S, *et al.* Identification of *DIO2* as a new susceptibility locus for symptomatic osteoarthritis. Hum Mol Genet 2008; 17(12): 1867-75. [http://dx.doi.org/10.1093/hmg/ddn082] [PMID: 18334578]

[27]   Daans M, Luyten FP, Lories RJU. *GDF5* deficiency in mice is associated with instability-driven joint damage, gait and subchondral bone changes. Ann Rheum Dis 2011; 70(1): 208-13. [http://dx.doi.org/10.1136/ard.2010.134619] [PMID: 20805298]

[28]   Hashimoto K, Oreffo RO, Gibson MB, Goldring MB, Roach HI. DNA demethylation at specific CpG sites in the IL1B promoter in response to inflammatory cytokines in human articular chondrocytes. Arthritis Rheum 2009; 60(11): 3303-13. [http://dx.doi.org/10.1002/art.24882] [PMID: 19877066]

[29]   Bagis S, Sahin G, Yapici Y, Cimen OB, Erdogan C. The effect of hand osteoarthritis on grip and pinch strength and hand function in postmenopausal women. Clin Rheumatol 2003; 22(6): 420-4. [http://dx.doi.org/10.1007/s10067-003-0792-4] [PMID: 14677019]

[30]   Bedson J, Croft PR. The discordance between clinical and radiographic knee osteoarthritis: a systematic search and summary of the literature. BMC Musculoskelet Disord 2008; 9: 116-22.

[http://dx.doi.org/10.1186/1471-2474-9-116] [PMID: 18764949]

[31]   Chan WP, Huang GS, Hsu SM, Chang YC, Ho WP. Radiographic joint space narrowing in osteoarthritis of the knee: relationship to meniscal tears and duration of pain. Skeletal Radiol 2008; 37(10): 917-22.
[http://dx.doi.org/10.1007/s00256-008-0530-8] [PMID: 18594811]

[32]   Calvo E, Palacios I, Delgado E, *et al.* High-resolution MRI detects cartilage swelling at the early stages of experimental osteoarthritis. Osteoarthritis Cartilage 2001; 9(5): 463-72.
[http://dx.doi.org/10.1053/joca.2001.0413] [PMID: 11467895]

[33]   Menashe L, Hirko K, Losina E, *et al.* The diagnostic performance of MRI in osteoarthritis: a systematic review and meta-analysis. Osteoarthritis Cartilage 2012; 20(1): 13-21.
[http://dx.doi.org/10.1016/j.joca.2011.10.003] [PMID: 22044841]

[34]   Spector TD, Cicuttini F, Baker J, Loughlin J, Hart D. Genetic influences on osteoarthritis in women: a twin study. BMJ 1996; 312(7036): 940-3.
[http://dx.doi.org/10.1136/bmj.312.7036.940] [PMID: 8616305]

[35]   Zhang W, Doherty M, Leeb BF, *et al.* EULAR evidence-based recommendations for the diagnosis of hand osteoarthritis: report of a task force of ESCISIT. Ann Rheum Dis 2009; 68(1): 8-17.
[http://dx.doi.org/10.1136/ard.2007.084772] [PMID: 18250111]

[36]   Kloppenburg M, Kwok WY. Hand osteoarthritis-a heterogeneous disorder. Nat Rev Rheumatol 2011; 8(1): 22-31.
[http://dx.doi.org/10.1038/nrrheum.2011.170] [PMID: 22105244]

[37]   Bijsterbosch J, Visser W, Kroon HM, *et al.* Thumb base involvement in symptomatic hand osteoarthritis is associated with more pain and functional disability. Ann Rheum Dis 2010; 69(3): 585-7.
[http://dx.doi.org/10.1136/ard.2009.104562] [PMID: 20124359]

[38]   Zhang W, Nuki G, Moskowitz RW, *et al.* OARSI recommendations for the management of hip and knee osteoarthritis: part III: Changes in evidence following systematic cumulative update of research published through January 2009. Osteoarthritis Cartilage 2010; 18(4): 476-99.
[http://dx.doi.org/10.1016/j.joca.2010.01.013] [PMID: 20170770]

[39]   Turcot K, Armand S, Lübbeke A, Fritschy D, Hoffmeyer P, Suvà D. Does knee alignment influence gait in patients with severe knee osteoarthritis? Clin Biomech (Bristol, Avon) 2013; 28(1): 34-9.
[http://dx.doi.org/10.1016/j.clinbiomech.2012.09.004] [PMID: 23063098]

[40]   Osteoarthritis: care and management/ Guidance and guidelines/NICE https://www.nice.org.uk/guidance/cg177

SUBJECT INDEX

A

ACE inhibitors 79, 123, 134, 137, 138, 139
Acetaminophen 190, 202
Acid 18, 173
  5-aminosalicylic 18
  folic 18
  inosic 173
Acidosis, renal tubular 91, 97, 101
Activated partial thromboplastin time (APTT)
  81
Activated RASFs 9
Activators, plasminogen 193
Acute cutaneous lupus 73
Acute gout 175
Adalimumab 19, 61
Adipokines 8, 195
Aggrecan 191, 193, 194
Aggrecanases 191, 193
Alcohol consumption 171, 174, 175
Aldolase 108, 112
Allergic rhinitis 90, 103, 143, 163, 164
Allopurinol 171, 181, 182, 183, 184, 187
Allopurinol and febuxostat 182, 184
Allopurinol dose 183, 184
Alternating buttock pain 29
Alveolar haemorrhage 159, 161, 164
Alveolitis 132
American College of Rheumatology (ACR)
  11, 70, 92, 124, 147, 149, 151, 159, 165,
  167, 176
Amino acid sequence 2, 30
Amyloidosis, secondary 15, 62
Amyopathic dermatomyositis 117
Anaemia 71, 156
Anakinra 61, 180
Analgesics 40, 70, 203
ANCA-associated vasculitis (AAV) 144, 155
Anemia 18, 20, 98, 116
Aneurysms 146, 148, 150, 153, 155, 169
Ankylosing spondylitis 27, 28, 29, 31, 33, 37,
  38, 56

juvenile onset 27, 28
Ankylosing spondylitis activity score (ASAS)
  35, 38, 44
Ankylosing spondylitis disease activity score
  (ASDAS) 34, 35
Ankylosis, early 37
Anterior ischemic optic neuropathy (AION)
  149
Anterior uveitis 27, 29, 42, 55, 58, 62, 168
Antibodies 67, 68, 81, 82, 123, 128, 134, 143,
  144
  anticentromere 123, 128
  cytoplasmic 134, 143, 144
Anticardiolipin 67, 68, 81, 82
Anticardiolipin antibodies 81, 84
Anti citrullinated peptide antibodies (ACPA)
  1, 3, 5, 9, 10, 11, 12
Antineutrophil cytoplasmic antibodies
  (ANCA) 134, 144, 155, 156, 157
Antinuclear antibodies 73, 77, 98, 112
Antiphospholipid antibodies 67, 68, 70, 77,
  81, 83, 85
Anti-RNA polymerase III 125
Anti-RNA polymerases II and III antibodies
  123
Anti-Scl-70 antibodies 123, 128
Arginine residues 5
Arterial hypertension, pulmonary 123, 124,
  125, 126, 127, 132
Arteritis, giant cell 143, 144, 146, 147, 148
Arthritis 1, 11, 12, 13, 27, 28, 31, 32, 33, 41,
  42, 43, 47, 50, 51, 52, 53, 54, 55, 56, 58,
  59, 60, 61, 62, 63, 69, 72, 76, 77, 97,
  123, 135, 138, 153, 156, 164, 167, 172,
  184, 190, 191, 197, 199
  asymmetrical 54, 56
  chronic 27, 28, 52, 54
  common type of 190, 191
  disease-associated 52
  disease-related 27
  enthesitis-related 50, 53, 56
  erosive 1, 12

www.ingramcontent.com/pod-product-compliance
Lightning Source LLC
Chambersburg PA
CBHW050832220326
41598CB00006B/357